SPORTS NUTRITION
FOR YOUNG ADULTS

SPORTS NUTRITION FOR YOUNG ADULTS

A Game-Winning Guide to Maximize Performance

JACKIE SLOMIN, MS, RDN

ROCKRIDGE PRESS

For general information on our other products and services or to obtain technical support, please contact our Customer Care Department within the U.S. at (866) 744-2665, or outside the U.S. at (510) 253-0500.

Rockridge Press publishes its books in a variety of electronic and print formats. Some content that appears in print may not be available in electronic books, and vice versa.

Interior and Cover Designer: Sean Doyle

Photo Art Director/Art Manager: Tom Hood

Editor: Gurvinder Gandu

Production Editor: Ashley Polikoff

Photography © Shutterstock/LanaSweet, cover; iStock/Chet_W, cover and pp. ii, 53, 105, 163; iStock/AlexRaths, cover; iStock/marilyna, p. 46; iStock/happy_lark, p. 54; iStock/AndreyPopov p. 66; iStock/skodonnell p. 80; iStock/Foxys_forest_manufacture, p. 98; iStock/Eugeniusz Dudzinski, p. 106; iStock/bhofack2 p. 128; iStock/porosolka, p. 142; iStock/Prostock-Studio, p. 156.

ISBN: Print 978-1-64611-709-3 | eBook 978-1-64611-710-9

R0

For my dad, who taught me to be relentless about pursuing my dreams, even if he doesn't realize it. Thank you for always believing in me.

CONTENTS

INTRODUCTION

HEY. MY NAME IS JACKIE. I'm a sports dietitian and fueling expert who helps young adults improve their performance and health by showing them how to make simple changes in their food and nutrition. As a private-practice dietitian with 10-plus years of schooling who has worked with hundreds of high school- and college-aged athletes, I've made it my mission to show active individuals how they can perform better, recover faster, and gain a competitive edge on and off the field. I've dreamed of being a dietitian since I was eighteen years old and first discovered how incredibly different I felt after changing my eating habits. Throughout my teenage life I was constantly exhausted and grumpy without even realizing that how I felt wasn't right. I thought feeling tired was normal and that everyone felt like I did. During my first year of college, my roommate introduced me to the basics of nutrition, training, and healthy eating. I became obsessed with nutrition and learned everything I possibly could on how to properly fuel my body, so I could feel and perform my best every single day. From that moment on, I knew the rest of my life was meant to be spent helping other athletes and active young adults reach their performance goals and improve their lives in the process.

Whether you're a long-distance runner looking to improve endurance or finish times, a gymnast looking to better your core strength, or a wrestler looking to make weight, having a performance fueling plan is the key to reaching your goals and to helping dedicated athletes transform into champions.

So how does a growing athlete go about implementing a fueling plan to gain a competitive edge? It can be challenging at first. Youths and young-adult athletes are in a very unique situation. Not only is your body naturally growing, giving you greater energy (calorie) and nutrient requirements compared to an adult, but also you have much greater needs because of the training intensity and additional strains put on the body from the extra hours of practice each week. A young athlete's energy needs could be double those of the average adult. But with a bit of planning, it can be easy to come up with a fueling strategy to maximize performance.

To have a successful performance fueling plan, there are three key components that you need to take into account: (1) the nutrient quality of the foods you're eating, (2) the frequency and specific timing of meals and snacks around practices or games, and (3) proper hydration. Nutrient quality refers to how nutritious and beneficial a certain food is to the body based on its overall composition and energy/nutrient density. Timing and frequency of foods plays a dramatic role in how much energy athletes have during activities, how quickly they recover, and even in how quickly they're able to build strength and muscle mass. And last but not least is hydration. Most athletes know hydration is important, but they don't know exactly how or why. Proper hydration can be the difference between getting burned out and fatigued halfway through a match or being able to dominate the field the entire game. Together, these three components will be your secret weapons in gaining a competitive edge.

PART I

The Nutritional Needs of Young-Adult Athletes

NUTRITION IS THE PROCESS OF CONSUMING the proper amount of nourishment and energy, and it includes two groups of nutrients. Energy-yielding nutrients, sometimes called macronutrients, include protein, carbohydrates, and fat, all of which come from a variety of food and fluids. Within those macronutrients are other components called micronutrients. These consists of vitamins, minerals, and phytochemicals.

Just like a team needs all of its players working together to accomplish a goal, these components have different but equally important roles in the body, and you need all of them working together, in the right amounts, to maintain optimal health. As an athlete, your goal is to get a balanced and large variety of all different types of nutrients in addition to making sure your total calorie (energy) intake is enough to support growth, training, and recovery.

As stated earlier, the nutrition needs of young-adult athletes can be double those of an older athlete because their bodies are undergoing some amazing changes. The body is creating new bone, tissue, and skin every time a growth spurt happens, on top of supporting training, recovery, and the production of new muscle mass. It's no wonder that the body has some serious energy and nutrient needs. Most young adults need to take in an additional 500 to 750 calories per day compared to their adult counterparts.

The truth is, all athletes are practicing and training on a regular basis, but not enough players are using their secret weapon: nutrition. If you want to get a competitive edge, then a proper nutrition strategy has to be part of your playbook.

CHAPTER ONE

THE NUTRITION LINEUP

EVERYTHING AN ATHLETE EATS AFFECTS THEIR BODY in a positive or negative manner, and in turn, affects their performance. Consuming the right balance of macro- and micronutrients is key. In the macronutrients category, protein is the basic building block of muscle and strength improvement. If your goal is to increase power or dominate the field, then getting the right amount of protein can be a game changer in how quickly you see strength gains. Next, carbohydrates are the body's main fuel source and are necessary for balancing energy throughout the day. Strategically fueling with carbohydrates, especially before and during practices or games, will help your fuel tank stay at 100 percent no matter how long you've been playing. And last, fat is necessary for supporting brain function, storing energy, and helping to absorb other nutrients.

As for micronutrients, vitamins, minerals, and phytochemicals are your support system. Everything from energy production, strength gains, and even recovery time is impacted by whether you're getting the right nutrients in your diet. Much like a team on the field, you need *all* different types and amounts of nutrients to work in unison in order to achieve peak performance. If you're a quarterback on a football team, for instance, it doesn't matter how great your pass completion rate is if the rest of the team isn't able to pull their weight. You can only be successful by working together. Nutrition works in the same exact way.

THE STARTERS: ENERGY-YIELDING NUTRIENTS

In order for champions to properly fuel their bodies, they need to consume the right amount and combination of energy-yielding nutrients in order to sustain activity, encourage recovery, and promote muscle growth during and after training. The three energy-yielding nutrients that the body requires are carbohydrates, protein, and fat. These nutrients contain energy in the form of calories, and all are major players in terms of their ability to help an athlete fuel properly and break performance barriers. Your energy needs as an athlete are much higher than a typical individual's because of the additional strain from training and practice that the body undergoes on a regular basis. For most healthy, active individuals, the daily calories needed will typically fall into the following ranges, depending on your specific sport or goal: from carbohydrates: 45 to 65 percent; from protein: 10 to 35 percent; and from fat: 20 to 35 percent.

In some cases, though, energy needs will vary from what is listed above. Individuals who have food sensitivities or allergies to specific foods like dairy or gluten, or those who have certain conditions that affect the body's ability to metabolize certain nutrients, such as diabetics, will have their own unique energy recommendations in order to optimize performance. Special diet considerations when determining energy needs will be addressed later in this book.

CARBOHYDRATES

Carbohydrates are like an athlete's secret weapon. This powerhouse nutrient contains four calories per gram and is the main fuel source for any type of moderate to intense activity. In other words, during any practice, training, or match, your body predominantly uses carbohydrates to fuel your muscles and brain. If you've ever forgotten to eat before an important game and felt like you were gassing out, fatigued, or unable to think clearly, it could have been from a lack of energy from carbohydrates. Now, the good thing about this all-star nutrient is that carbohydrates can either be broken down immediately into glucose and used for energy, or stored in the body as glycogen via the muscles or liver for use at a later time. In other words, if we choose the right carbohydrate sources we can keep our energy topped off at all times and play our hardest when it counts.

So how do we know how much and what type of carbohydrates to choose? Carbohydrates actually come from a very wide variety of foods, but their main two forms are called simple carbohydrates and complex carbohydrates. The main difference between these two types of carbohydrates is how long it takes the body to break them down.

Simple Carbohydrates

Simple carbohydrates consist of foods that are very easy for the body to break down, and they provide a rapid form of energy to the body for a shorter period of time. They can come from foods that have natural sugar, such as fruits and vegetables, but the biggest source of simple carbohydrates in most American diets comes from foods that have a large amount of added sugars, such as baked goods, desserts, and sugar-sweetened beverages.

Simple carbohydrates can be a smart fuel choice in certain instances. Since simple carbs are broken down quickly and we gain access to the energy almost immediately, they're an excellent choice to eat if your meal or pre-workout snack is going to be within one to two hours of a training or practice and you want to get immediate energy to your muscles and brain. You also want to consume simple carbohydrates right after activity as part of a post-workout meal or snack, so the body can get an immediate fuel source to replenish energy stores. The quicker your body gets access to carbohydrates and glucose, the faster you'll be feeling 100 percent again and the faster you'll recover from your workout or activity. This goes for both endurance- and strength-related sports.

In these instances, try to get most of your simple carbohydrates from natural, whole foods instead of processed foods with added sugar, as the latter typically contain large amounts of unwanted calories. Not only are processed foods less nutritious, but they often won't leave an athlete feeling satiated, and you may find yourself feeling hungry quickly. You may also have a quick boost of energy followed by a bout of fatigue soon after eating them.

Simple carbohydrate sources:

- Cake
- Candy
- Cookies
- Fruit
- Milk
- Pie
- Soda
- Sports Drinks
- Syrup
- Yogurt

Complex Carbohydrates

Unlike simple carbs, complex carbohydrates take the body a moderate amount of time to break down since they require more work. This means you're going to be fueling your body and providing steady energy for several hours. So what's the main difference between complex carbohydrates and simple? In addition to providing sustained energy, complex carbohydrates can also be rich in other extremely important components, such as fiber, vitamins, minerals, antioxidants, and phytochemicals. The last four all play an important role in keeping the body healthy and keeping you at peak performance, but one component in particular deserves to be in the spotlight, and that is dietary fiber. Fiber actually slows down the digestion of food in the body. This is a great thing, because that means foods rich in fiber will provide a steadier and longer form of energy without potential crashes. Additionally, you're less likely to overeat or consume larger-than-average portion sizes when your carbohydrate sources are complex because you'll feel satiated faster.

Much like simple carbohydrates, not all complex carbs are created equal. You want to get the majority of your complex carbohydrates from whole-grain sources instead of processed foods. Whole-grain choices are packed with fiber, vitamins, minerals, antioxidants, and phytochemicals; processed complex carbohydrates, such as white breads and some pastas, have had most of the nutrients and fiber stripped away from them. In other words, do your best to choose whole-grain and whole-wheat products to get the most benefit.

The extra components in complex carbohydrates help maintain energy levels, shorten recovery time, and even keep the body feeling fuller for longer. Foods such as whole-grain breads or pasta, legumes, and vegetables all fall into the category of complex carbohydrates, and in general, we want most of our carbohydrates to come from these types of foods. All the extra bonuses that are bundled together with complex carbohydrates mean that they pack a punch in making sure we're getting exactly what our bodies need on and off the field.

Complex carbohydrate sources:

- Beans
- Bread
- Butternut Squash
- Corn
- Couscous
- Lentils
- Oats and Oatmeal
- Peas
- Potatoes
- Pumpkin
- Quinoa
- Rice
- Sweet Potatoes
- Whole-Grain Pasta

Carbohydrate Requirements

Carbohydrate needs vary greatly among athletes, depending on age, gender, current weight, and weight goals in addition to the length and intensity of an average practice or game. While it would be impossible to give an exact number, the following directions can be used to determine your estimated carbohydrate needs for the entire day.

STEP ONE: Determine your weight in kilograms (kg). We will be using kilograms to calculate all energy and calorie needs, so we need to convert to that from your weight in pounds. To do this, divide your current body weight in pounds by 2.2 to get your weight in kilograms. As an example, if you weigh 150 pounds:

- 150 lbs / 2.2 = 68 kg

STEP TWO: Determine your carbohydrate needs based on your estimated training intensity:

Light intensity: Your workouts are less than one hour per day and are primarily strength-based, or are a mix of cardio (jogging, running, calisthenics), strength, and/or technique work.

- Carbohydrate needs based on light intensity workouts: 4 to 5 grams of carbohydrates per kilogram of body weight

Medium intensity: Your workouts are approximately one hour per day and are primarily strength-based, or are a mix of cardio, strength, and/or technique work.

- Carbohydrate needs based on medium intensity workouts: 6 to 7 grams of carbohydrates per kilogram of body weight

High intensity: Your workouts are greater than one hour per day and are primarily cardio but may contain a small amount of strength and/or technique work.

- Carbohydrate needs for high intensity workouts: 7 to 8 grams of carbohydrates per kilogram of body weight

STEP THREE: Calculate your range of carbohydrate needs based on your estimated training needs. For example, if you weigh 150 pounds, and you fall into the medium intensity category, multiply your weight in kilograms (68 kg) by each range: Weight (kg) x carbohydrate needs (g) = daily carbohydrate needs (g)

- Lower range: 68 kg x 6 g = 408 g
- Higher range: 68 kg x 7 g = 476 g

So, our 150-pound athlete's estimated carbohydrate needs for the day are 408 to 476 grams of carbohydrates.

PROTEIN

When most athletes think of what type of fuel they need to gain a competitive edge, it's usually copious amounts of protein. This isn't surprising, since most gyms and online sites touting fitness advertise products such as protein bars and powders that have 25 or even 50 grams of protein in them per serving. The general thought is that more is always better, but if you want to be competitive it's important to understand how much protein the body actually needs for a competitive edge and how much is a detriment.

Protein is needed for building and repairing muscles after exercise, and it's an essential component in many other functions of the body, including the production and maintenance of skin, hair, nails, and hormones. Protein carries vitamins throughout the body for absorption and helps keep our immune system up and running. In short, protein provides the building blocks for a wide variety of functions in the body.

Much like carbohydrates, protein can be broken down into different classifications. Protein is actually made up of components called amino acids, of which there are more than 20 different kinds. While some amino acids can be produced in the body, others that are considered essential must come from food sources. Foods that are rich in essential amino acids and are considered high-quality sources of protein come predominantly from animal products, including poultry, meat, fish, eggs, yogurt, milk, and cheese. Additionally, there are many plant-based sources of protein that contain amino acids. Good sources of plant-based protein include items such as beans, legumes, nuts, nut butters, seeds, whole-grain bread and pasta, and vegetables. Ideally, you want to get a mix of animal and plant-based proteins to meet your protein needs so that your diet is rich in a variety of different foods.

Now, here are some words of wisdom to ensure you're fueling for success: Believe it or not, most athletes naturally meet their protein needs throughout the day. Despite this, many still go above and beyond what their needs are, because they believe consuming more will make them stronger and provide a competitive edge. This is often done by cutting out carbohydrates to make room for more protein-rich foods and even extra-protein supplements. But this type of plan actually sets up athletes for failure instead of success.

As mentioned earlier, the body's main fuel source for activity is carbohydrates. But our body is also very, very adaptable. When we cut carbohydrates to make room for more protein, our body will actually convert some of the extra protein we're eating into carbohydrates for energy! Not only that, our body requires synergy in order to fuel optimally and feel its best. And this goes for consuming a proper ratio of carbohydrates to protein. For example, after a training or game the body requires foods that are rich in carbohydrates in order to help transport protein to the muscles to aid in recovery.

So how much protein does the average athlete need? Much like carbohydrate needs, an athlete's protein needs are going to depend on age, growth rate, training demands, and sport type. Use the following directions to calculate your estimated protein needs.

STEP ONE: Determine your needs based on your body composition goals:

If your goal is to MAINTAIN your current strength or muscle mass and MAINTAIN OR INCREASE your weight, then your estimated needs are

* 1.2 to 1.4 grams of protein per kilogram of body weight.

If your goal is to IMPROVE your strength and muscle mass and MAINTAIN OR INCREASE your weight, then your estimated needs are

* 1.5 to 1.7 grams of protein per kilogram of body weight.

If your goal is to MAINTAIN your current strength and LOSE weight, then your estimated needs are

- 1.7 to 2.0 grams of protein per kilogram of body weight. Protein needs become higher during weight loss to help preserve lean muscle mass.

STEP TWO: Calculate your range of protein needs based on your body composition goals. Take your weight in kilograms (page 5) and multiply it based on the numbers determined in step one. For example, if a 150-pound athlete wants to improve strength and maintain weight, then we'll calculate protein needs based on the range of 1.5 to 1.7 grams:

- Lower range: 68 kg x 1.5 g = 102 g
- Higher range: 68 kg x 1.7 g = 116 g

Tip: Just eating protein isn't enough to build strength and muscle mass. You need to regularly engage in resistance- or strength-training workouts that exhaust your muscles in order for protein to do its job and rebuild them stronger than before.

FAT

Fat is an incredibly important yet often misunderstood nutrient for athletes. Most individuals think all fat is bad and want to keep the amount of fat in their diet as low as possible. The truth, though, is that dietary fat plays a huge role in overall health and yes, you guessed it, athletic performance. Dietary fat is responsible for optimal brain function, helps the body absorb certain vitamins and nutrients, protects your organs, and even helps with thermoregulation. We'll discuss thermoregulation and how it affects performance in the hydration section of this chapter (page 16). And while dietary fat may not be the optimal fuel source for your average training or game day, it is a main fuel source for low-intensity activity such as walking. This means that fat still plays an important role in keeping your energy balanced throughout the day.

There are a few different types of fat—those we want our diet rich in, as they provide many health benefits, and others that we may want to limit, as they can cause inflammation or other health issues if consumed too often. Fats found in most animal products, such as poultry, beef, pork, milk, butter, and other dairy products, are called saturated fats. These types of fat are solid at room temperature and promote inflammation in the body if consumed in large quantities. Trans fat is another type of fat we want to limit in our diet. Trans fats are actually artificially created and are typically found in baked goods, such as pastries, pies, cookies, dough, and fried foods.

The types of fat we predominantly want to consume in our diet are the two types of unsaturated fats: monounsaturated and polyunsaturated fats. Unsaturated fats are actually anti-inflammatory and have been shown to improve cholesterol levels. Unsaturated fats can be found in foods like nuts, nut butters, avocado, seeds, and fatty fish such as salmon, tuna, and sardines.

So how do we determine how much fat should be in our diet? Calculating fat needs can be a bit more difficult than determining protein or carbohydrate needs. The reason is that protein and carbohydrate needs are directly based on how active you are or what your strength goals are. Fat, however, is calculated based on a specific percentage of total calories in the diet. So, to determine fat needs, first we need to calculate how many calories you're likely burning throughout the day. While there are a multitude of different ways to calculate an athlete's calorie needs, we're going to use a simple and easy-to-calculate method to get our answer.

STEP ONE: Calculate your baseline calorie needs. To determine estimated calorie needs, multiply your weight in kilograms (page 5) by 24 to get your base calorie needs. As an example, if you're a 150-pound athlete (150 lbs / 2.2 = 68 kg):

- 68 kg x 24 = 1600 calories

Once we have this number, we need to multiply it based on your level of physical activity throughout the day to get your total estimated needs.

STEP TWO: Calculate your total calorie needs. Take your baseline calorie needs and multiply it based on which category your training intensity falls into. This should match the same training intensity you chose when calculating carbohydrate needs (page 6):

- Light intensity: multiply your baseline needs by 1.3 to 1.4
- Moderate intensity: multiply your baseline needs by 1.5 to 1.6
- Heavy intensity: multiply your baseline needs by 1.7 to 1.8

For example, if we go back to our 150-pound athlete who had a moderate training intensity:

- Lower range of calorie needs: 1600 x 1.5 = 2400 calories
- Higher range of calorie needs: 1600 x 1.6 = 2560 calories

This individual's estimated calorie range is 2400 to 2550 calories per day to maintain his weight.

STEP THREE: Determine the calories from fat needs. As a rule of thumb, you want your calories from fat to be between 25 and 35 percent of your total calorie needs for the day. To calculate your total calories that will come from fat, we can simply multiply your daily estimated calorie needs by 0.25 and 0.35 to get your range. In our example, total daily calories are 2400 to 2560, so we'll use 2500 to have a nice, even number for our calculations.

- Lower range: 2500 calories x 0.25 = 625 calories
- Higher range: 2500 calories x 0.35 = 875 calories
- Total daily calories from fat = 625 to 875 calories per day

STEP FOUR: Determine the number of grams of fat per day. Our final step is to convert your calories of fat into grams. Because each gram of fat is approximately 9 calories, we simply divide your calories from fat by 9 to get our estimated needs in grams. For example:

- Lower range: 625 calories per day / 9 = 69 grams of fat
- Higher range: 875 calories per day / 9 = 97 grams of fat
- Total estimated grams of fat per day: 69 to 97 grams

THE ROLE PLAYERS: MICRONUTRIENTS

If macronutrients are the starting lineup of the team, micronutrients would be considered its role players. While micronutrients don't provide energy or calories, they do contain other compounds that are arguably just as important. Micronutrients consist of vitamins and minerals, and your body relies on them for everything from proper energy production, immune system boosts, and even mood regulation. Even a non-athlete has to get an adequate number of micronutrients to feel healthy. Just as young athletes have increased energy and calorie needs, they also have increased needs for certain vitamins and minerals and are more prone to deficiencies. Being deficient in just one vitamin or mineral might not seem like a big deal, but it can have an astronomical effect on your performance. A vitamin deficiency could be the difference between a fatigue-related injury or even the match-winning point.

VITAMINS

In general, vitamins are classified into two different categories: water-soluble and fat-soluble. Water-soluble vitamins cannot be stored in the body if you consume more than your body can absorb at any one time. Any extra water-soluble vitamins are excreted in urine. This is why taking a multivitamin that has a much higher percentage of your daily needs for any particular vitamin can cause your urine to have a dark yellow color and odor. It's simply the body getting rid of extra vitamins it cannot use. Water-soluble vitamins include various B vitamins as well as vitamin C. On the other end of the spectrum are fat-soluble vitamins. Fat-soluble vitamins can be stored in the body in fat cells. Fat-soluble vitamins include vitamins A, E, D, and K.

While all vitamins and minerals are important for the body to function optimally, there are specific ones that hold greater significance.

Vitamin A

Vitamin A is a fat-soluble vitamin whose most well-known role is in promoting healthy vision and eyesight. For athletes, however, vitamin A has another extremely important function: acting as an antioxidant. Antioxidants are especially helpful to the body during times of intense stress, such as during intense training sessions. Vitamin A can predominantly be found in dark leafy greens such as broccoli, spinach, and collard greens, as well as in carrots, sweet potatoes, eggs, milk, and fortified cereals or grains.

Vitamin B6

Vitamin B6, also known as pyridoxine, is a water-soluble B vitamin that plays a critical role in the metabolism of carbohydrates, and to a lesser degree, protein and fat metabolism. In other words, if you don't have enough B6, your body won't be able to properly create these key energy sources, and you may suffer from fatigue on and off the field. While vitamin B6 cannot be produced in the body and must come from food sources, it is actually found in a wide variety of common foods, including meat, fish, poultry, pork, eggs, fortified grains, and vegetables.

Vitamin B12

Vitamin B12, also known as cobalamin, is another water-soluble vitamin in the B family. Vitamin B12 plays a critical role in energy production and is involved in the production of red blood cells. Too little B12 can have detrimental effects on athletic performance. A B12 deficiency causes megaloblastic anemia, which may cause chronic fatigue, delayed recovery, and even difficulty with split-second decision-making during a game. B12 deficiencies are actually relatively common, as B12 can only be consumed in the diet, specifically from animal products such as meat, poultry, fish, eggs, milk, yogurt, and fortified grains. This makes vegetarians and vegans who do not consume animal products especially prone to B12 deficiency. Many vegan and vegetarian products, such as plant-based milks, soy, and some breakfast cereals, are therefore fortified with B12 to help aid in proper consumption.

Vitamin D

Vitamin D, also called cholecalciferol, is a fat-soluble vitamin of special importance because it has such a huge array of roles in the body. Vitamin D is involved in maintaining bone health, a strong immune system, proper blood sugar and energy levels, cardiovascular health, and mood. Vitamin D can actually be a tricky vitamin to get in the diet as it doesn't have many food sources, but it can be found in fatty fish such as salmon and tuna, fortified milk, cereal, eggs, and orange juice. Luckily, this vitamin also comes from sunlight, so if you play an outdoor sport or spend a few minutes in the sun each day, you can improve your vitamin D levels. Be aware of the symptoms of a vitamin D deficiency. Bone fractures, especially stress fractures, can become common in those with a deficiency, as well as muscle weakness, fatigue, delayed recovery time, and depression. These are definitely not symptoms we want if our goal is to maximize our performance while staying healthy.

Vitamin Recommendations for Males

AGE RANGE	VITAMIN A	VITAMIN B6	VITAMIN B12	VITAMIN D
14 to 18	900 ug/d	1.3 mg/d	2.4 ug/d	15 ug/d
19 to 25	900 ug/d	1.3 mg/d	2.4 ug/d	15 ug/d

Vitamin Recommendations for Females

AGE RANGE	VITAMIN A	VITAMIN B6	VITAMIN B12	VITAMIN D
14 to 18	700 ug/d	1.2 mg/d	2.4 ug/d	15 ug/d
19 to 25	700 ug/d	1.3 mg/d	2.4 ug/d	15 ug/d

MINERALS

Iron

Iron is a mineral that plays an important role in an athlete's health. Iron helps transport oxygen throughout the body and is necessary in order for the body to have proper energy stores. Without enough iron and, thus, oxygen, individuals will suffer from fatigue, brain fog, a lowered immune system, and decreased physical performance. A deficiency in iron can eventually transform into anemia as well, further exasperating these symptoms. Women are more prone to iron deficiencies than men due to menstrual blood loss, but all players should ensure they're meeting their iron needs through their diet. Foods rich in iron are beans, nuts, spinach, fortified cereals and grains, meat, and clams.

Calcium

Calcium is a mineral with a synergistic relationship to vitamin D. Both are needed together to maintain proper bone health and avoid fractures, which is why most foods fortified with vitamin D will also be fortified with calcium. Additionally, calcium is responsible for muscle contractions during daily activities as well as during training and competition. Calcium deficiencies can lead to fatigue, muscle cramps, and irregular heart beat, in addition to raising the risk for brittle bones and fractures. Luckily, calcium is found in most dairy products, including milk, cheese, and yogurt, as well as in dark leafy greens, dried fruits, and tofu.

Sodium

Sodium is unique in the fact that it's not only a mineral, but also a major electrolyte whose main role is to regulate the body's fluids and blood pressure. Sodium often gets a bad rap since the average individual who eats out will often encounter very large amounts of sodium in their diet. But sodium plays a particularly important role for those who are active or engaging in sports. When the body has too much sodium, it will hold on to additional fluids in the body. This is why individuals can often feel bloated or puffy after eating a very salty food. On the other hand, too little sodium in the body leads to something called hyponatremia (too little salt), which can cause headaches, confusion, nausea, or vomiting—this is especially common in endurance athletes. Active young adults need to pay special attention to sodium levels as they lose large amounts of sodium and potassium when sweating. (This is why most sports drinks contain electrolytes, in order to replace what may have been lost in sweat. We'll discuss those later when we look at hydration.) In addition to sports drinks, sodium can be found in items like salted pretzels, salted nuts, pickles, and most frozen or canned goods. High sodium levels are also found in highly processed foods such as fast food, but should generally be limited due to the high-calorie, high-saturated-fat, and low-nutrient profile of these foods.

Potassium

Much like sodium, potassium is a mineral and electrolyte involved in fluid regulation as well as muscle contractions and blood pressure. Potassium can often be found alongside sodium in sports drinks, but can also be found naturally in foods such as bananas, oranges and citrus fruits, cantaloupe, honeydew, apricots, potatoes, watermelon, coconut water, and many other fruits and vegetables.

Mineral Recommendations for Males*

AGE RANGE	IRON	CALCIUM	SODIUM	POTASSIUM
14 to 18	11 mg/d	1300 mg/d	1500 mg/d	4700 mg/d
19 to 25	8 mg/d	1000 mg/d	1500 mg/d	4700 mg/d

Vitamin Recommendations for Females*

AGE RANGE	IRON	CALCIUM	SODIUM	POTASSIUM
14 to 18	15 mg/d	1300 mg/d	1500 mg/d	4700 mg/d
19 to 25	18 mg/d	1000 mg/d	1500 mg/d	4700 mg/d

Vitamin and mineral needs are based on the average, sedentary population. While there are no specific guidelines for athletes, nutrition needs may be greater due to additional caloric and physical demands during physical exercise.

The Scoop on Polyphenols

Polyphenols are unique micronutrients that are found naturally in plant foods, including a large variety of fruits and vegetables. While they are not quite the same as vitamins, they have a few amazing benefits for athletes. Polyphenols help with digestion and decrease the risk of certain diseases, but are best known for their antioxidant properties, which can help fight inflammation in the body. By nature, most athletes will build up inflammation after a training, practice, or game. This is typically recognized as soreness. Polyphenols can help combat that inflammation and, if your diet is rich in them, may be able to help speed up your recovery time and get you back on the field or into the workout room faster. One important distinction to make, however, is that not all polyphenols are created equal, so it's important to know where you're getting your source from. Polyphenols found naturally in foods are completely safe and have the health benefits touted above, but this isn't the case with supplements. When buying a supplement that contains polyphenols, you may be consuming 500, 1,000, or even 10,000 times the amount that is found naturally in food. Ironically, when you consume too many polyphenols, they actually have the opposite effect on an athlete and become pro-inflammatory instead, which can hinder recovery time. This is why it's best to stick with natural sources. Foods rich in polyphenols include apples, berries, grapes, spinach, broccoli, carrots, and dark chocolate.

THE MVP: HYDRATION

While macronutrients and micronutrients all have an indispensable role in an athlete's performance and health, hydration is actually the most important factor for sustaining peak performance. Picture fluids as the glue that holds your entire team together: the team captain, if you will. Your hydration level directly affects all other functions in the body, so it's extremely important to make sure your fluids are topped off for peak performance. Hydration actually plays a role in distributing nutrients, oxygen, and hormones throughout the body and helps with digestion, and keeping joints lubricated. Proper fluid intake allows us to keep our mind sharp, avoid fatigue, and keep our heart rate steady during rest and competitions. Hydration also plays a huge role in thermoregulation, which is the process of keeping your body's core temperature in the right range. Just like a phone or computer, if your temperature isn't regulated properly you may begin to overheat, which will have a drastic effect not only on your performance, but also your overall health.

ELECTROLYTES

It's hard to talk about hydration without mentioning electrolytes! Electrolytes are a special type of mineral that comes from food and certain beverages and that helps regulate hydration in the body. We actually lose electrolytes when we sweat as part of the body's mechanism to regulate temperature, so during periods of training greater than one hour and especially for endurance athletes, it is especially important to replace electrolytes. Losing too many electrolytes can result in dehydration, irregular fluid balance, and even cramping or nausea. Some of the most important electrolytes to focus on for performance are sodium, chloride, and potassium.

Sodium

Sodium is the most critical electrolyte that regulates water in the body, both in and around cells. Of all the electrolytes, sodium is lost most rapidly during extended periods of activity. Food sources of sodium for athletes include salted pretzels, pickles, and rice cakes.

Chloride

Chloride is the second-most-abundant electrolyte to be lost during activity. It's typically lost alongside sodium, though in slightly lesser amounts. In addition to helping with fluid regulation, chloride also helps maintain the body's pH and blood pressure. Because chloride is often found right alongside sodium, any food rich in sodium will also likely be rich in chloride.

Potassium

Just like sodium and chloride, potassium helps regulate fluids, but it has an additional role in helping with muscle contractions to prevent cramping and maintain heart rhythm. Foods rich in potassium include bananas, oranges and citrus fruits, cantaloupe, honey, and potatoes.

Electrolyte Recommendations for Males*

AGE RANGE	SODIUM	POTASSIUM	CHLORIDE
14 to 18	1500 mg/d	4700 mg/d	2300 mg/d
19 to 25	1500 mg/d	4700 mg/d	2300 mg/d

Electrolyte Recommendations for Females*

AGE RANGE	SODIUM	POTASSIUM	CHLORIDE
14 to 18	1500 mg/d	4700 mg/d	2300 mg/d
19 to 25	1500 mg/d	4700 mg/d	2300 mg/d

Electrolyte recommendations are based off of the average, sedentary population. While there are no specific guidelines for athletes, needs may be higher due to increased perspiration during physical activity.

FLUID DEPLETION

Most athletes think of "sweat" when they think of how the body loses fluids. But there are actually a number of ways the body naturally loses fluid throughout the day, both at rest and during physically activity. By nature, your body can lose several ounces or even gallons of fluid a day, which is excreted through urine and feces. You also lose fluids naturally through skin ventilation and while breathing. Fluids are even lost during metabolism, when the body is breaking down food into nutrients. These processes are completely normal and are used as a mechanism to continuously balance fluid and keep your body's temperature exactly where it needs to be. During physical activity, of course, you lose additional fluid in a much more rapid manner through sweating. Even a young adult's environment plays a big role in the amount of fluids lost throughout the day. Athletes who live in hot and humid environments or who work out in extreme cold, live at a high altitude, or wear many layers of clothing or equipment are all prone to having greater fluid losses both on and off the field. Fluid loss can cause anything from a slightly increased heart rate and fatigue to more serious signs and symptoms of dehydration such as nausea, cramping, or even heat-related illnesses. It's important to make sure the body is constantly being hydrated throughout the day.

FLUID INTAKE

Luckily, there are plenty of easy ways to consistently take in hydration to combat the body's natural loss of fluid throughout the day and during practice. The most obvious and simple method is to continuously drink fluids. While water is the main fluid most athletes think of, and likely the one that should be consumed in the greatest quantity, all beverages count as fluid and will help keep you hydrated. This means items like sports drinks, juice, milk or chocolate milk, and herbal tea can all help replace fluids the body is losing. Sports drinks with added sugars have a place in an athlete's diet during prolonged physical activity, but aren't necessary during non-exercise times. More information on sports drinks and when to choose the appropriate type can be found in chapter 15 (page 157). It should be noted, however, that beverages with caffeine cause extra fluid loss, so drinks like coffee or caffeinated tea won't help as much.

What might not be as well known is that many foods have an extremely high water content and will also keep you hydrated. Most fruits and some vegetables are actually predominantly made of water. Foods with the highest water content include watermelon, cucumbers, cantaloupe, strawberries, tomatoes, and celery. Getting a mix of fluids and foods with a high water content will go a long way in keeping fluids topped off, which will help keep you in a state of balance (homeostasis) and allow you to perform your best both mentally and physically.

DEHYDRATION

There is no doubt that dehydration can ruin an athlete's performance faster than any other cause, and it can often strike before you're even aware. When someone "feels" thirsty, they're often already dehydrated and suffering from the physical and mental side effects even if they're not aware. Even losing 1 or 2 percent of total body weight in water can lead to athletes having trouble concentrating not only on the field, but also throughout the day, such as in class or while studying. Dehydration also causes a young adult's body temperature and heart rate to rise, since it's missing the additional fluid it needs to cool itself off. For every liter of fluid the body loses, your heart rate increases by approximately 8 beats per minute. Not only does the body have to work harder during any activity, but your rate of perceived exertion increases. This is a term that means that physical activity feels more strenuous than it actually is. Running feels more difficult, your endurance capacity is lowered, and you may even struggle to do basic exercises or technique training that is normally second nature. When the body loses even more of its total water, about 3 to 5 percent, dehydration symptoms become more serious and will turn into muscle cramps, nausea, vomiting, diarrhea, or even heat stroke. While it's not extremely common, severe dehydration—losing 8 to 9 percent of your total water—can even result in fatality.

The best way to avoid dehydration is to proactively come up with a fluid plan based on an individual's unique sweat rate and fluid loss. It's also important to consistently check your hydration status throughout the day. Some people sweat an average amount, while others are considered "heavy sweaters." This means not only do they lose fluids more quickly, but they may also be losing a larger amount of electrolytes in their sweat. An easy way to check if you are a heavy sweater or not is to see if there is residue on your skin after a heavy practice. If there is a slightly white or grainy residue on the skin, this is actually a buildup of sodium and electrolytes that have been lost through perspiration. A good rule of thumb to check overall hydration status is to see what color your urine is. Ideally, you want your urine to be a very pale yellow, almost like lemonade. This likely signifies good hydration and means you're on the right track. If a young adult's urine is a much darker or amber color, similar to apple juice, it means the body has likely not gotten enough fluids throughout the day. The chart on the following page can be used to assess current hydration status based on urine color.

Urine color and hydration status

COLOR	HYDRATION STATUS
	Pale yellow to clear = well hydrated
	Light yellow = ideal hydration
	Moderate yellow = okay but rehydration needed
	Yellow and cloudy = not great; rehydration necessary
	Dark yellow/amber = slightly dehydrated
	Dark or orange tint = severely dehydrated

CHAPTER TWO

THE BUILDING BLOCKS OF A HIGH-ENERGY DIET

WOULD YOU RATHER PLAY A GAME OF CARDS BLINDFOLDED or while wearing a pair of X-ray glasses? Most people would pick the glasses. Understanding what nutrition an individual should be fueling with to get the best possible performance boost comes down to a similar choice. When athletes understand exactly what foods and drinks are best for their bodies, they stack their odds of getting the best nutrition possible, so they can play their hardest and give it their all without playing a guessing game with their fueling choices. In this chapter, we're going to discuss exactly what should be taken into consideration when making food and drink choices in order to give a young-adult athlete the best possible advantage.

DRINK CONSIDERATIONS

As discussed in the previous chapter, hydration is one of the most important factors for a young adult, especially those looking to operate at peak performance. Getting the right amount and types of fluid will allow you to maintain your energy level throughout the day, avoid brain fog, and make sure your body doesn't overheat. So, what exactly should young adults be drinking to stay properly hydrated? With so many different beverages on the market, your options are limitless. But there are a few common drink choices that pop up more than the rest for young adults. While these may be popular options, some are more beneficial than others for performance and energy.

WATER

For those who regularly exercise fewer than 60 minutes per day, water alone is enough to rehydrate the body properly. It doesn't have added sugars or other mystery ingredients like many beverage options on the market. However, for those who engage in longer physical activity, an electrolyte beverage may be a better option.

Water comes in many different packages and varieties that are processed in different ways. Tap water is perhaps the most common and includes all water sources in a building or home. Tap water is typically safe to drink; occasionally, however, this water can be contaminated with lead or other substances if there is a pipe leak. One benefit of tap water is that it contains minerals, including calcium, magnesium, potassium, sodium, and phosphorous, many of which are important electrolytes for hydration or to help support healthy growth.

Filtered water is tap water that has been purified by using a small chemical or physical barrier. While this does get rid of contaminants, it may also remove minerals, depending on the type of filter used. Bottled water can come from a variety of sources such as lakes and glaciers, but many bottled water brands are simply filtered tap water that has been packaged in plastic. Sparkling water, also called club soda, is water that has had carbon dioxide added to it in order to create carbonation. While carbonated water doesn't directly impact hydration, some individuals have reported drinking less due to feeling fuller faster when drinking carbonated beverages. Like all other water sources, the amount of minerals and potential contamination will depend on where the water is sourced from and what the filtering process is like.

SPORTS DRINKS

Sports drinks often contain a combination of fluids, quick-digesting carbohydrates, and electrolytes to promote hydration. Such drinks can be a great option for those who are exercising more than 60 minutes or for endurance athletes, but aren't typically needed otherwise. Many commercial sports drinks also contain ingredients like high-fructose corn syrup or artificial dyes, so it's important to choose a quality drink or make your own. For specific recipes and tips on how to make your own sports drink, refer to chapter 15 (page 157).

MILK

Milk is a fluid choice that not only hydrates, but also contains quick-digesting carbohydrates, protein, and certain vitamins and minerals like calcium and phosphorous. Milk or other dairy products should be consumed 2 to 3 times per day; however, too much can increase daily calorie consumption considerably. Some individuals may experience stomach upset when consuming milk or other dairy right before physical activity, so it's best to test this out before adding it to your pre-workout fuel.

Whole milk is cow's milk that has not had any of the fat content removed. While all dairy-based milk contains quick-digesting carbohydrates and roughly 8 grams of protein per cup, whole milk is higher in saturated fat and calories. While you want to limit the overall amount of saturated fat in the diet, whole milk can be part of a balanced diet and contains plenty of nutrition packed in a glass, including calcium and vitamin D.

Low-fat milk is cow's milk that has undergone a process to remove some of the fat content that is naturally present. The amount of protein and carbohydrates in a cup is exactly the same as whole milk, but it may have up to 75 percent less fat and one-third fewer calories than whole milk.

Chocolate milk is cow's milk that has had chocolate syrup or other types of sugar, cocoa, and/or artificial flavorings added to give it a flavor. Chocolate milk can either be whole milk, low-fat, or fat-free depending on how it's been made, so the nutrient profile can vary greatly.

Nut milks are often preferred by individuals who are lactose intolerant or have a dairy allergy. They can come from a variety of different sources, but the most common are almond, coconut, cashew, and hazelnut. Nut milk is made by soaking nuts in water for an extended period of time, blending the nuts and

Tips to Prevent Heat-Related Health Issues

Fluid-related issues that occur from being in extreme heat or cold:

- Nausea
- Vomiting
- Diarrhea
- Cramping
- Brain fog
- Higher heart rate
- Increased rate of perceived exertion

Tip 1: Begin your day by giving your body a fluid boost. Aim for at least 8 fluid ounces or 1 cup of water first thing in the morning to kick-start your fluid goals.

Tip 2: Invest in a reusable water bottle to carry around throughout the day. Even taking small sips at regular intervals can add up to some big improvements in your hydration.

Tip 3: Don't wait until you feel thirsty to begin drinking more fluids. Thirst is a sign of dehydration, which means you're already feeling the effects even if you don't realize it.

Tip 4: Eat water-loaded fruits and veggies. Raw fruits and vegetables are predominantly made up of water and are a great way to supplement your fluid intake.

Tip 5: Add a flavor to your water if you're struggling to drink just plain water. Mixing it up by adding a small amount of fruit juice or a natural flavor can help increase fluid consumption.

Tip 6: Drink plenty of fluids before, during, and after every practice. If possible, try to take small sips from your water bottle every 15 minutes. If your practice doesn't make that feasible, be sure to make a point to get in plenty of water right after practice.

Tip 7: Consider an electrolyte beverage or foods that have sodium, chloride, and potassium in addition to your water if your practice regularly lasts an hour or longer, or if you're a heavy sweater.

water together, and then straining the residue out to produce a beverage. The main difference between nut milk and cow's milk is that nut milk is often much lower in protein. Also, the nutrient profile of this beverage can vary greatly depending on the process used to make the drink.

FRUIT JUICE

Fruit juice contains a mixture of fluids, vitamins, minerals, and quick-digesting carbohydrates. Much like milk, the nutritional benefits of fruit juice can vary greatly depending on what's in it and how much is being consumed. Some juices will advertise that they are made with 100 percent fruit, while others may be only 10 percent or even 1 percent juice with the rest being a mixture of water, sugar (or artificial sweetener), and other varying ingredients. Small amounts of fruit juice can be beneficial, but since most juices contain no fiber, they are calorie-dense options that will typically not keep you satiated for long compared to consuming a piece of whole fruit. Fruit juice by itself may not be the best beverage choice during physical activity depending on the product. High concentrations of carbohydrates and sugar in fruit juice can cause cramping in some individuals, so it's best to stick with a different refueling option when possible.

ENERGY DRINKS

Energy drinks have dramatically increased in popularity over the last few years, especially with young adults and athletes. Often touting benefits like increased energy, they may be a go-to choice before practice. Unfortunately, energy drinks come with many potential risks. Most energy drinks contain large amounts of caffeine: between 80 and 200 milligrams, which is the equivalent of 1 or 2 cups of coffee. Additionally, these products often contain large amounts of B vitamins, some with 500 percent or even 10,000 percent of the recommended daily dose, as well as herbal supplements like guarana and ginseng, which are considered stimulants. Unfortunately, the mix of all of these ingredients together can result in increased anxiousness, nervousness, mood swings, and even depression.

Sports drinks often get lumped in with energy drinks, but most sports drinks don't contain caffeine or herbal supplements. If you're choosing a refueling beverage, it's advisable to go with a sports drink rather than an energy drink.

PROTEIN SHAKES

Depending on the brand and type of shake, protein shakes can be an excellent source of protein and fluids throughout the day. Shakes may be beneficial for a select few who struggle to get in their daily protein needs, but are likely not needed for most young adults who have a balanced diet.

COFFEE AND TEA

It can be tempting for young-adult athletes to reach for a caffeinated drink such as coffee or tea to help them stay up to study or cram for a test after a long day of practice. A cup of coffee typically has between 80 and 100 milligrams of caffeine in it, but many places offer cup sizes that are double or even triple that size. Tea typically has a much lower caffeine content, with the average cup yielding between 40 and 80 milligrams of caffeine, and herbal tea contains no caffeine at all. Caffeine has been shown to reduce fatigue and make exercise feel easier, particularly with endurance sports. However, it should be noted that caffeinated beverages do affect every individual differently. While some people may feel more energetic, others may get anxious or jittery. These side effects become more prevalent with larger amounts of caffeine intake. The National Collegiate Athletic Association lists caffeine in large quantities as a banned substance, with a urinary caffeine concentration of 15 micrograms per millimeter (roughly 500 milligrams) resulting in a positive drug test. You would need to consume roughly 6 to 8 cups of coffee 2 to 3 hours before a competition to reach these levels, but athletes should be aware of the risks.

A note about specialty coffee drinks: While these drinks technically do contain fluids, they're often packed full of added sugars. To top it off, caffeinated beverages act as diuretics, which means they may make you excrete even more fluid throughout the day.

ALCOHOL

While alcohol should never be consumed by young adults under the age of 21, it can be a popular choice among athletes of legal age. Unfortunately, there is a large cultural tradition drinking after a particularly difficult game, or socially at dinner or on weekends. However, alcohol consumption can seriously impact your performance. Alcohol is a depressant, so it slows down reaction speed and motor function, and inhibits proper balance. Drinking can also affect sleep quality, resulting in a more fatigued and miserable athlete at practice the next day. On top of performance deficits, alcohol is a significant source of calories with the average beer containing 150 to 200 calories per bottle. Alcohol also displaces the absorption of many B vitamins, meaning those who drink regularly are more at risk for vitamin deficiencies, which can lead to symptoms such as depression and chronic fatigue. It's best for athletes to avoid drinking the night before a practice or game and to practice moderation at other times if they engage in alcohol consumption in general.

How to Decipher Nutritional Labels

Knowing how to read a nutritional label can be one of the best tools for young adults to use to make healthy choices that will benefit their performance and body composition goals. Use these tips to pick the best options:

1. Always check the portion size of an item at the top of the label. Without looking, you could be eating 3 or even 4 servings in a container without realizing it.

2. If selecting a snack or drink for fuel pre-workout, post-workout, or during exercise, try to stick with options that have less than 200 calories per serving, less than 5 grams of fat, and less than 2 grams of fiber.

3. Try to choose minimally processed foods and stick with short ingredient lists when possible. A common misconception is that if you can't pronounce an ingredient, then it is automatically harmful. While this is not always the case, there is a grain of truth to this concept when it comes to specific ingredients. If possible, avoid foods with the following ingredients in them:

   Fats and trans fats: hydrogenated or partially hydrogenated oils, palm oil, shortening

   Sugars and sweeteners: sugar, sucralose, aspartame, corn syrup, high-fructose corn syrup, maltodextrin, saccharin

   Added preservatives and flavorings: sodium nitrite, sodium nitrate, monosodium glutamate or MSG

   Dyes: Red, blue, green, yellow

4. Look for foods with less than 10 grams of added sugar per serving and more than 3 grams of fiber per serving, except right before a match or practice. An exception can be made for high-sugar items like fruits, which are nutrient-rich, high in fiber, and contain phytochemicals.

FOOD CONSIDERATIONS

With all of the different food choices out there, it's easy to be confused about what should be in a balanced diet for a young adult. While everyone's needs may vary slightly, there are some general guidelines you can use to build performance-winning plates that are both delicious and healthy. A diet rich in whole foods with minimally processed ingredients will have the most benefits. You want to build plates that are rich in fruits, vegetables, whole grains, protein (particularly lean protein), and dairy. Fruits, vegetables, and whole grains are nutrient powerhouses that will help keep you energized, full, and feeling your best, while lean protein will support your muscle growth and recovery. Dairy provides a mix of carbohydrates and protein as well as important nutrients like calcium and vitamin D, which is important for building strong bones and keeping your mood regulated.

FRUITS

Fruits sometimes get a bad rap because of the confusion about sugar content. But fruits are jam-packed with several B vitamins; minerals such as iron, magnesium, potassium, and phosphorous; antioxidants; and phytochemicals. Fruits are predominantly made up of carbohydrates and can either be low or high in fiber, making them a great choice whether you need a low-fiber option before a game or a high-fiber option throughout the day. Low-fiber fruits include bananas, watermelon, and nectarines, while some high-fiber options are mangoes, strawberries, and raspberries. Besides their health benefits, fruits can be one of the easiest portable snacks to pack if you're low on time. It doesn't get much easier than tossing a banana or apple in your bag to munch on while running to practice. Fruits are also considered low-energy dense foods, which is a phrase meaning they're typically low in calories. Fresh and frozen fruits typically contain the most nutrients, but canned fruits in water can be a good option if nothing else is available. Dried fruits also have many benefits, but keep in mind they have a much lower water content and are often much more calorie-, sugar-, and fiber-dense per ounce than fresh alternatives. With the serving size of fruit being one cup raw (about one medium fruit) or one-half cup cooked, it's actually pretty easy to get in the recommendation of at least 2 to 3 servings per day.

VEGETABLES

Like fruits, vegetables are also chock-full of nutrients and chemicals your body needs to thrive. They are rich in things like vitamin C, vitamin A, and folic acid. Vegetables can be non-starchy foods like tomatoes, peppers, and dark leafy greens, which are low-energy dense foods; or starches such as potatoes, sweet potatoes, corn, peas, and beans, which are considered high-energy dense. A high-energy dense food is one that is rich in calories per serving. As an example, an energy-dense starch can have double or triple the calories of a non-starchy vegetable serving. Like fruits, most vegetables are primarily carbohydrate based; however, foods such as beans and chickpeas can also be a good vegetarian protein source. Starchy foods typically take longer to break down in the body and are a good choice to eat in moderation throughout the day to keep your energy levels balanced and avoid a crash. Just like fruits, the serving size for vegetables is one cup raw or one-half cup cooked, and you want to aim for at least 2 to 3 servings per day. While making cooked veggies could be fast or complicated depending on the recipe, tossing some baby carrots or celery sticks in your bag is an easy way to hit your veggie goals for the day.

WHOLE GRAINS

Whole grains are an excellent source of energy and nutrition for any athlete's plate. Whole-grain carbohydrate sources are foods that are either unprocessed or only processed a small amount. This means that these foods are great sources of vitamins—especially B vitamins—fiber, and of course, carbohydrates. Many people have the misconception that whole grains (and grains in general) cause weight gain, but typically the cause is actually excess caloric intake that comes with foods that accompany whole grains, such as butter, oil, and cheese. Whole grains, like other carbohydrate sources, help keep you fueled for activities, balance your energy throughout the day, keep you satiated, and keep your bathroom trips regular. Examples of whole-grain foods include whole-grain and whole-wheat pastas and bread, brown rice, and barley. The main reason you want to choose whole grains over refined grains such as white bread or white rice is that when these foods are processed, they're often stripped of the vitamins, minerals, antioxidants, fiber, and other important compounds that keep your body operating at its best. There isn't necessarily a specific daily serving size that fits everyone since each athlete will have different calorie needs, but try to make sure at least 50 percent of your intake consists of whole grains.

DAIRY

Dairy products are foods derived from animal milk. The most common dairy foods are milk, cheese, and yogurt. So, should dairy be a regular part of your diet? For those without lactose intolerance or a food allergy to milk-derived products, dairy should definitely be a regular part of your diet. Dairy products contain beneficial vitamins and minerals such as calcium, vitamin D, and phosphorous, which help athletes build strong bones and support performance. Additionally, dairy provides a combination of all three energy-yielding nutrients (protein, carbohydrates, and fat), depending on the fat content of the product you're buying. Full-fat products such as whole milk or cheese have greater amounts of saturated fat, while low-fat or skim-milk products have had some or all of the fat removed from them. Both types can fit well into a young adult's diet, and it will often come down to personal preference and timing to decide which choice is best. Of note, when consuming low-fat or skim-milk products, it's beneficial to check the ingredient list on the label, as some products will replace the fat content with added sugars. The serving size for milk is one cup; for cheese is one ounce; and for yogurt is six ounces or three-quarters cup. Ideally, you want to consume 2 to 3 servings of dairy per day to meet your calcium needs.

MEAT AND EGGS

When most young adults think of protein sources, they think of meat. Meat consists of red meat (beef, venison, pork, lamb), poultry (chicken, turkey, duck), and seafood (fish, shellfish). Additionally, eggs are a non-flesh animal product that is a protein source. Meat and eggs are an excellent source of protein, containing seven grams per one ounce cooked, but the fat content between these animal products varies greatly depending on the type. Red meat and dark meat in poultry all contain large amounts of saturated fat, which is pro-inflammatory and can cause other health problems if eaten in excess over time. All food is fine in moderation, but in order to be at peak health and performance, you want the majority of your meats to be lean protein sources such as chicken and turkey.

One food that should be emphasized despite being considered "fatty" is fatty fish, such as white tuna or salmon. While the fat content in these foods is higher, fatty fish are rich in a component called omega-3 fatty acids. Omega-3 fatty acids are anti-inflammatory and help promote recovery, mood, and overall health. Since omega-3 fatty acids can't be made in the body, it is recommended to aim for at least 2 servings of fish per week in order to get enough. The recommended serving size of animal protein is three ounces of cooked meat (four ounces raw) per day.

BUILDING A GAME-CHANGING DIET PLAN

The foods you eat and drink every single day have the biggest impact on your performance, but fueling for the day of training or competition is also extremely important. What you eat before, during, and after training will vary based on the exact time you're fueling as well as the type of training and intensity of your sport. This is because it takes longer for some foods to digest than others. Part two of this book will go more in-depth into nutrient timing and how to apply it to your own training and competition days. If your pre-workout or pre-competition meal is 2 or 3 hours before training, it's perfectly okay to have a regular, balanced meal that contains protein, carbohydrates, fat, and fiber. However, the closer you get to game time, the less fat, fiber, and protein you want to consume, as these foods can take longer to digest, sit "heavy" in the stomach, and make you feel sluggish while trying to perform physical activity. If you're eating within 1 to 2 hours of practice or competition, choose foods low in fat and fiber and limit protein, or else you'll slow your digestion too much and you won't get the energy you need. In this case, aim to consume 0 to 1 serving of protein, 1 to 2 servings of carbohydrates, and 0 to 1 serving of fat. If you're not able to eat until right before your training or competition and are getting your fuel source in less than 60 minutes beforehand, you only want to consume 1 to 2 servings of low-fiber, quick-digesting carbohydrates and as little protein and fat as possible to ensure you get that immediate energy boost! During training, aim to get in four ounces of water after every 15 minutes of activity. If your training or competitions consistently go for an hour or longer, swap out the water for a sports drink. After training or practice, it's important to get in a combination of quick-digesting carbohydrates to replenish energy stores, and lean protein to facilitate muscle recovery and growth.

2 to 3 hours before training

CARBOHYDRATES: 45–65%	PROTEIN: 10–35%	FAT: 20–35%

½ cup cooked old-fashioned or steel cut oatmeal with:

1 tsp honey

1 tbsp nut butter

½ banana or 1 cup strawberries

1 scrambled or hardboiled egg

16 fl oz (2 cups) water

1 to 2 hours before training

CARBOHYDRATES: 70–80%	PROTEIN: 20–25%	FAT: 0–5%

½ turkey or chicken sandwich on whole-wheat bread:

1 slice whole-wheat or whole-grain bread

2+ slices tomato + lettuce

2 oz lean turkey or chicken

1 tbsp light mayonnaise

1 medium apple or ½ large banana

8 fl oz (1 cup) water

0 to 1 hour before training

CARBOHYDRATES: 100%

1 banana, medium

or

16 fl oz sports drink

4 to 8 fl oz (½ to 1 cup) water

During training

CARBOHYDRATES: 0 OR 100%

Training < 60 minutes: 4 fl oz water every 15 minutes

Training > 60 minutes: 4 fl oz sports drink every 15 minutes

0 to 1 hour after training

CARBOHYDRATES: 70–80%	PROTEIN: 20–25%	FAT: 0–5%
2 oz tuna or chicken packed in water 12 saltine crackers		
1 to 1½ cups water for every pound of weight lost during training*		

To determine fluid needs after training, weigh yourself before and after practice. For every 1 pound lost, aim to get in 16 to 24 fluid ounces (1 to 1½ cups) of water

Pro(tein) Tips

Believe it or not, most young adults are able to get in their daily protein needs by simply consuming a balanced diet containing all of the food groups previously listed. One of the easiest ways to ensure adequate protein intake is to set a goal to consume the appropriate daily servings of protein and dairy throughout the day. Including a protein source at every meal, whether it be dairy, meat, or plant-based, will go a long way toward reaching your goals. For example, having a Greek yogurt in the morning with scrambled eggs and toast will already put you around 20 grams of protein at breakfast. For lunch and dinner, try including lean proteins such as chicken, turkey, or fish in your sandwiches, soups, or salads for a quick protein boost. A three-ounce serving of cooked lean protein provides 21 grams of protein and is only about the size of a deck of cards! Plant-based protein is also an excellent way to help meet your daily needs, while also getting extra vitamins, minerals, and fiber. Try adding beans, nut butters, lentils, edamame, or tofu to your meals for an extra protein and nutrient boost. A half-cup serving of cooked beans contains about 7 grams of protein, while a half-cup of tofu includes 10 grams.

SPECIALTY DIETS

While it is entirely possible for young adults to get the right amount of nutrients (including energy-yielding nutrients and micronutrients) from food alone, certain individuals who follow special diets or have food restrictions are at a higher risk for having nutrient deficiencies. This is because most popular diets end up limiting or eliminating one or more of the major food groups that you get your nutrition from. Luckily, with some smart planning, you can still set up your diet and nutrition plan for success to make sure you're fueling adequately no matter what your specific diet is.

VEGETARIAN

Vegetarians are individuals who consume a plant-based diet and have eliminated eating any meat. People choose to become a vegetarian for many reasons: They believe a predominantly plant-based diet is healthier than eating meat; they do not like the way animals are treated in our food supply chain and have decided not to participate in the buying or consumption of meat; or they believe a vegetarian diet will help facilitate weight loss. While there are many variables regarding each of these circumstances, it's important to respect someone's decision to be vegetarian regardless. With the removal of meat from the diet, it can be easy to assume that all vegetarians are going to be short on their daily protein requirements and will need to consume supplements. There are, however, a number of sources of both plant-based and dairy-based foods that are rich in protein. Vegetarians can look to the following food choices for substitutes to animal proteins that will help them meet their needs: beans, legumes, tofu, tempeh, edamame, milk, cheese, yogurt, eggs, quinoa, nuts, and nut butters.

VEGAN

While similar to vegetarians, vegans choose not to consume both meat and foods that are made from animal products. This means foods like milk, cheese, yogurt, and even honey in some cases are off-limits in the diet. Individuals following a vegan diet have a higher risk for being deficient in certain nutrients, particularly vitamin B12, iron, calcium, and vitamin D. Vitamin B12 is found almost exclusively in animal products, while calcium and vitamin D are typically found in dairy. There are a handful of plant-based sources of vitamin D, calcium, iron, and B12 that should be planned into the diet. Plant sources of calcium include foods like fortified plant-based milks, fortified orange juice, cooked spinach, tofu, soybeans, legumes, and enriched breads and whole grains. Vitamin D can be found in fortified plant-based milks, fortified orange juice, and tofu, or obtained via daily exposure to sunlight. Vegan-friendly foods with vitamin B12 include fortified grains as well as nutritional yeast. Note that nutritional yeast has a cheese-like flavor and is a wonderful substitute to put on salads, pasta dishes, or even in dressing. For those who are having a particularly difficult time incorporating these foods into their diet, it may be necessary to take a daily multivitamin to ensure adequate nutrient intake.

GLUTEN-FREE

Young adults following a gluten-free diet typically have an intolerance or allergy to the protein found in gluten and can experience an array of nasty symptoms if they accidentally consume a gluten-containing food. Symptoms may include nausea, vomiting, cramping, or even acne breakouts and can last for hours, days, or weeks. This is why it's especially important for those following a gluten-free diet to make sure they're eating the right foods. Being on a gluten-free diet typically restricts an individual's food choices in the supermarket and while eating out. Because almost all grains naturally have gluten in them, these individuals must avoid all breads, pasta, rice, baked goods, cereals, and desserts that are not exclusively listed as being gluten-free on the label (typically signified with a GF symbol or Gluten-Free on the packaging). Additionally, those who are gluten-free also must check food labels to ensure that what they're buying wasn't manufactured on shared equipment. Even though items like oats, barley, and rye may not trigger someone's gluten sensitivity, these items are commonly made on shared equipment and may be contaminated. Always check the back of your food label for a gluten-free symbol and for manufacturer claims on how the product was created. Those following a gluten-free diet may be at risk for deficiencies in B vitamins or have a diet low in carbohydrates due to the avoidance of grains. This is because gluten-free products (even grains) are often not fortified with the same amount of B vitamins that their gluten-containing counterparts contain. Ensure that your diet is rich in plant sources of B vitamins such as vegetables, nuts, beans, seeds, and fruit for adequate nutrient and carbohydrate intake throughout the day.

KETO

A ketogenic diet has traditionally been used by health care professionals in the treatment of epilepsy in young adults. Over the last decade, however, a keto diet has become increasingly popular for those looking for weight loss or those who believe it has performance benefits. A true ketogenic diet has an extremely restrictive daily carbohydrate intake: typically fewer than 40 grams of carbohydrates on a daily basis. To put this into perspective, two slices of bread would put you near your carbohydrate limit for the day. A keto diet relies on consuming only protein and fat products such as animal protein and fats, cheese, and other sources of fat, including nuts and nut butters. The idea behind a keto diet is that an individual's body will adapt to using fat for fuel. While this concept holds some truth, it's important to understand the differences in energy production in the body, especially for an athlete. The body can in fact use fat as a fuel source, but as discussed earlier in this book, fat is not an efficient energy source for high-intensity activities such as a typical game, competition, or practice. The reason for this is because the body has a limit on how fast it can produce energy from fats. While some young adults report benefits from a keto diet, including increased energy and improved blood-health markers, others have reported the opposite, including extreme fatigue and depression. Because a ketogenic diet eliminates several foods groups, including grains, vegetables, and protein, it's important to give some serious thought to the pros, cons, and sustainability of this diet before starting it.

PALEO

The Paleo diet has also become popular in recent years. A Paleo diet, in simple terms, is a diet that is rich in animal protein, dairy, fruits, and vegetables, while eliminating all foods that contain grains. This means no cereal, rice, bread, pasta, baked goods, or desserts. Much like the other diets listed above, the Paleo diet eliminates an entire group of foods, which means there is the possibility for individuals to be at higher risk for certain nutrient deficiencies. Since most grains are fortified with B vitamins and calcium, it is important to ensure other sources of these nutrients are present in adequate amounts in the diet. Those following a Paleo diet should focus on filling their plate with a diverse mix of fruits, vegetables, legumes, nuts, and protein sources to satisfy nutrient requirements.

PART II

Nutrient Timing for the Win

AS A YOUNG-ADULT ATHLETE, you can improve strength and energy without any additional training simply by strategically incorporating certain fuel choices at specific times throughout the day. Luckily, this is entirely possible with something referred to as *nutrient timing*. The previous chapters discussed the impact of having a balanced diet throughout the day, and while this is important, it's not the only factor that matters. *When* you eat certain foods is just as important as *what* you eat. Nutrient timing is the intentional act of planning specific food sources around times of training and competition in order to maximize fuel, strength, and performance. Some foods digest rapidly and provide immediate energy, while others can take several hours to be broken down and, if not eaten soon enough before a competition, could lead an athlete to feel fatigued or sluggish. Understanding this concept could be the difference between performing below your capabilities and crushing the competition.

CHAPTER THREE

PRE-EXERCISE FUEL

OPTIMIZING YOUR DAY-TO-DAY NUTRITION should include strategically fueling before exercise. While you can't eat poorly on a daily basis and make up for it by having a good pre-exercise plan, you can and should be eating and drinking specific foods prior to activity to ensure maximal performance. How much a young adult should eat is determined by when they eat and what type of foods they can tolerate before activity.

THE BENEFITS OF FUELING BEFORE EXERCISE

Fueling before a training session or competition provides you with a competitive edge compared to an athlete running on an empty stomach. While every athlete will have different nutrition needs depending on the specific sport and activity intensity, most athletes will benefit from fueling before exercise for a number of reasons.

PREVENTS HYPOGLYCEMIA

Fueling properly before intense exercise will prevent something called hypoglycemia, which is a deficiency of blood sugar (glucose) in the body. Since carbohydrates (glucose) are an athlete's main energy source, it's important to keep blood sugar levels balanced throughout a competitive event or training to ensure an individual is able to perform.

FUELS MUSCLES

Your body also needs a pre-workout meal or snack to fuel your muscles during exercise. Without proper carbohydrate consumption, your body won't have the energy needed to utilize your strength properly.

IMPROVES REACTION TIME

Pre-workout energy does more than just fuel physical activity. It also helps fuel the brain and keep an active adult's senses sharp. Lack of fuel before activity could lead to brain fog or delayed reaction times.

MAINTAINS SATIETY

Arguably, nothing is more distracting on the field or court than trying to compete while hungry. Preemptively fueling before a long training session or competition can help athletes stay comfortably full and avoid mid-competition hunger.

WHAT TO EAT BEFORE EXERCISE

What each athlete or physically active young adult needs to eat before exercise depends not only on the type of exercise being done, but also on whether the sport is in or out of season. A gym enthusiast who works out 45 minutes a few times per week will have drastically different (and likely lower) needs than an athlete who is currently in season. Sport-specific recommendations for athletes will be covered later in this book. For the sake of this chapter, eating recommendations will be made with the assumption that those reading are currently in season and looking to maximize their training sessions or competition days. In addition, the type and amount of foods being eaten will vary depending on how soon food is being eaten before exercise. The longer the time period between eating and competing, the more balanced a meal can be with a combination of carbohydrates, protein, and fat. The closer an athlete is to competition, the more fuel choices should shift to low-fat and low-fiber, with a focus on carbohydrate choices that are easily digestible.

MEALS

Meals and pre-workout snacks will vary greatly, depending on how much time you have before activity to get fuel in. In addition to staying focused on hydration (refer to chapter 1, page 16, for recommendations), it's important to ensure that you're eating the appropriate foods so that your body has time to metabolize and absorb the fuel sources being provided.

If a practice or competition is 3 to 4 hours away, consuming a meal rich in carbohydrates with a moderate amount of protein and a healthy fat source is ideal. The specific amount of food needed will depend on your individual calorie and macronutrient requirements (page 5). Most young adults who are eating a full meal will need between 500 and 900 calories. Depending on how large a meal is and how many calories you are consuming, you may want to also eat a quick-digesting carbohydrate source fewer than 60 minutes before an activity to top off muscle glycogen and maximize energy.

Sample Meal Plan

	CARBO-HYDRATES	PROTEIN	FAT	CALORIES
Sandwich:				
2 slices whole-wheat bread	30g	4g	<1g	120
2 oz lean deli meat (turkey, ham, chicken)	-	14g	2g	60
Tomato	-	-	-	-
Lettuce	-	-	-	-
1 banana	30g	-	-	120
16 almonds, lightly salted	-	4g	10g	90
1 (6-oz) container low-fat yogurt	30g	7g	2g	160
Total:	90g	30g	14g	550

If your practice or competition is two to three hours away, the goal is still to focus on a carbohydrate-rich food source that is easily digestible, while also consuming a small-to-moderate amount of protein and fats. Since your body has less time to digest the food, it's recommended that you have a smaller meal than normal in order to avoid having partially digested foods sloshing around in the stomach. A good rule of thumb is to aim for 200 to 300 calories with 75 percent of your total fuel coming from a carbohydrate source.

Sample Meal Plan

	CARBO-HYDRATES	PROTEIN	FAT	CALORIES
½ sandwich:				
1 slice whole-wheat bread	15g	2g	<1g	60
1 oz lean deli meat (turkey, ham, chicken)	-	7g	1g	30
Tomato	-	-	-	-
Lettuce	-	-	-	-
1 banana	30g	-	-	120
8 almonds, lightly salted	-	2g	5g	45
Total:	45g	11g	6g	255

SNACKS

Athletes have many reasons to consume a pre-workout snack immediately before training or exercise: If your schedule doesn't allow you to eat until right before practice; if your game has been delayed and will put your last meal more than 4 hours before the start of your competition; or if you just need to top off glycogen stores before a particularly intense workout session. Since your body has very little time to digest food at this point, consuming only a small amount of quick-digesting carbohydrates with as little fat and protein as possible is recommended to avoid partially digested food in the stomach during activity. At this phase, most athletes want to focus on consuming 100 to 200 calories maximum and should choose carbohydrate sources with little or no fiber. Additionally, if you're an athlete with a sensitive stomach, a liquid fuel source may be better tolerated than a food source of carbohydrates.

Snack Suggestions (Pick One)

	CARBO-HYDRATES	PROTEIN	FAT	CALORIES
16 fl oz sports drink	40g	-	-	160
1 banana	30g	-	-	120
1.5 oz pretzels	30g	-	-	120
2 energy gels + 32 fl oz water	50g	-	-	200

Intermittent Fasting

As an athlete, you may have heard about the potential benefits of intermittent fasting. But what exactly is it? Intermittent fasting, often referred to as IF, is the act of voluntarily limiting your food consumption to a specific window of time during the day. Although there are many different types of intermittent fasting, the most common is the 16:8 method—16 hours of food restriction followed by an 8-hour window for consumption. Some research has shown that IF can help reduce body weight and body fat, lower cholesterol levels, improve satiety, and even reduce insulin resistance in certain individuals. However, this is not always the case. The main benefit of IF is in improving satiety in some individuals, which may lead to decreased caloric intake compared to those not undergoing IF. Despite this, there are also many challenges that you should be aware of if you're looking to try IF. Intermittent fasting can be severely restrictive to some individuals due to the strict "rules" around the times you can and cannot eat. Athletes may find that they have limited ability to control nutrient consumption during times of training and competition. If a practice isn't within your window of eating, then it becomes impossible to fuel properly for your activity, which can lead to fatigue, decreased endurance, and an overall performance decline.

WHAT TO DRINK BEFORE EXERCISE

What you drink before exercise has one of the biggest impacts on your ability to train and perform with maximal effort. As discussed in the previous chapter (page 22), hydration is directly linked to an athlete's performance and endurance capabilities. So, exactly how much fluid should an athlete be getting before a workout? Much like the food section of this guide, the amount of fluid you need depends on when your activity starts. Ideally, you should drink roughly eight fluid ounces (one cup) of water for every hour you're awake each day. This is simply to meet your basic needs and doesn't cover the additional fluids needed for training.

When you're two to three hours away from an activity, you should begin to ramp up your fluid intake to make sure you're properly hydrated going into a training or practice. Since you still have a couple hours at this point between hydrating and the actual activity, a simple water or a low-calorie beverage option will do. Drinking additional water at this point will allow it to be filtered through and excreted from the body prior to exercise. Once you get down to the one- to two-hour mark, you should revert back to eight fluid ounces to continue to have adequate hydration. (Remember that during the actual exercise, you're going to want to drink four ounces of liquids every 15 minutes.) If you are having a food-based pre-workout snack, then water or a low-calorie beverage option will work well. However, if you're someone who prefers to take in a liquid fuel source (fluids that contain calories and carbohydrates) then this fluid should be in the form of a sports drink, smoothie, or other liquid. These items can either bought or homemade (refer to the Homemade Sports Drink Recipes in chapter 15, page 157, for recipes and tips). If opting for a liquid fuel source, you will want to take in roughly 20 to 40 grams of quick-digesting carbohydrates at this time to top off glycogen stores and ensure you'll have adequate energy.

Hydration Schedule Before Competition

Morning or afternoon of competition	8 fl oz of water per hour
2 to 3 hours before competition	16 fl oz of water per hour
1 to 2 hours before competition	8 fl oz of water or a sports drink per hour

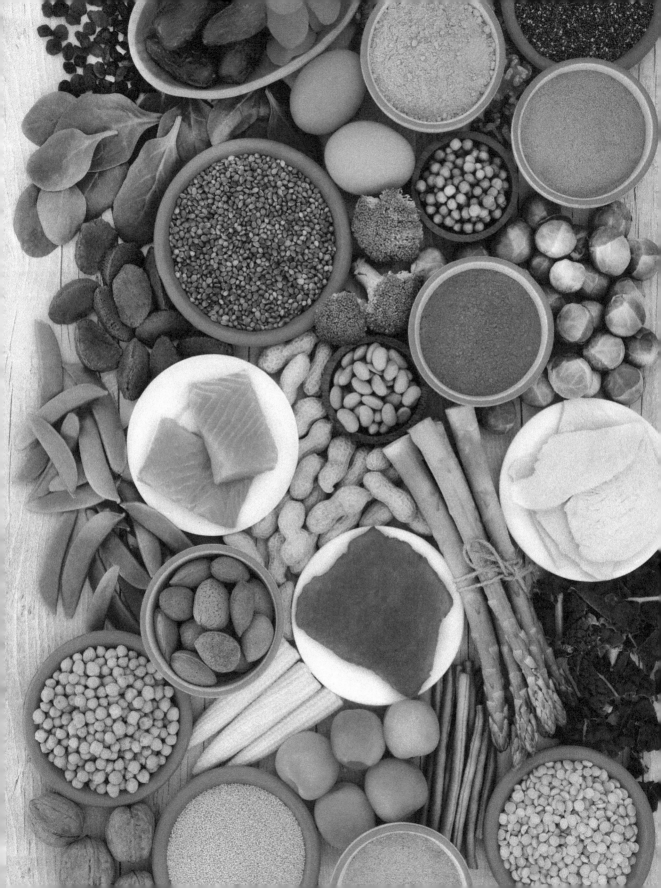

CHAPTER FOUR

EXERCISE FUEL

ALL THE PREPARATION IN THE WORLD for a big game or tournament will fall to the wayside if you're not fueling your body and muscles properly during the game as well. Between game day jitters, pregame training, or simply just being hyper-focused on your match, it's extremely easy for athletes to forget to fuel up in the middle of activity. The recommendations for fueling during exercise are extremely similar to those for before exercise. The goal is to top off muscle glycogen and avoid gastrointestinal (GI) distress so that you can maintain optimal energy levels and performance during the entire duration of activity. Athletes who don't top off their fuel sources are prone to fatigue and poor performance outcomes.

So, who should be eating during exercise, and what specifically should they be focusing on? All athletes and young adults who are practicing or competing in events lasting an hour or longer would likely benefit from a quick-digesting fuel source during exercise. There are a few things to keep in mind, though, when selecting the right fuel.

WHAT TO EAT DURING EXERCISE

Studies have shown that carbohydrate intake—particularly carbs that come from glucose and fructose—has the greatest impact on energy levels for athletes. Glucose is found in a wide variety of carbohydrate sources, while fructose is the type of sugar found specifically in fruits. Natural fructose is not the same as high-fructose corn syrup, an ingredient that is often found in processed foods and has been linked to insulin resistance and obesity. You want to make sure you're taking in the proper amount of each type of carbohydrate to get the best benefit.

Glucose and fructose work especially well together in the body, because they're absorbed using different pathways. This means that while your body can only process a certain amount of glucose per minute, it isn't limited on the amount of energy that can be supplied because it has an alternate means of getting energy via fructose. Having a food with a combination of glucose and fructose may increase energy availability by up to 50 percent.

On the flip side, you don't want to consume fructose alone or in very high amounts. Fructose alone can lead to GI upset or issues such as nausea and cramping.

Ideally, athletes should consume 30 to 60 grams of carbohydrates per hour in addition to fluids and electrolytes in order to replenish the glycogen being lost during activity. To put that into perspective, that is roughly 120 to 240 calories of quick-digesting carbohydrates every hour. Many athletes think these recommendations are only for endurance sports or for runners. However, research has shown that replenishing carbohydrates during activity also has a performance benefit for other sports such as wrestling, football, and lacrosse, which have staggered bouts of activity followed by periods of less activity or rest.

Choosing foods that are rich in both glucose and fructose, or foods that have a combination of different types of sugar, will have the best results and the least risk for GI distress. Many products on the market are formulated to contain the proper ratios of glucose to fructose and have been designed specifically with athletes in mind. Products like sports drinks, energy gels, and sports beans contain a mixture of glucose, fructose, electrolytes, and fluids. In the case of sports drinks, these products already contain the appropriate ratio of fluids to carbohydrates and electrolytes. Energy gels and sports beans, however, contain a concentrated amount of carbohydrates and electrolytes but do not have additional fluids. One common mistake athletes make is consuming these products without the necessary fluids, which will lead to negative GI symptoms. You certainly don't want to be in the middle of a race or a tied game and suddenly have to sprint off the field to the bathroom. If you're using gels or beans, be sure to get in 8 to 16 fluid ounces of water along with them and don't exceed the recommended portions.

Whether you're opting for a natural food source or a formulated sports product, never introduce a new food or fueling regimen before an important game or practice. All the research in the world can point toward what would likely work best for you, but every athlete's body is unique. While one person may feel like they have superhuman powers with a certain fuel, another may react poorly and end up in the outhouse instead of the outfield. The best time to try out a new food or fuel is always on a day off, or at the very least, during a practice that is not preceding an important game or competition.

Here are the steps to set up a fueling plan for exercise:

1. Determine if you will tolerate a food or fluid fuel source. For those who experience little to no stomach issues when eating right before or during practice, a solid food source is ideal. For those of you who do have a sensitive stomach or have difficulty tolerating food during physical activity, a purely liquid fuel source would be best.

2. Write down how long a practice or game will typically last. Are you going to be active for one hour or more?

3. Pick a food or fuel source you've previously tried out and determine the amount or number of serving sizes you'll need to stay fueled during the duration of your activity. Remember, you want to consume 30 to 60 grams of carbohydrates for every hour of activity.

4. Keep your surroundings in mind. If you don't have access to a cooler, choose shelf-stable foods or items that don't require refrigeration. If you only anticipate having a few minutes to get in your fuel during your match, it may be best to choose a liquid fuel source that's easily consumed in a short period of time.

Mid-Exercise Snack Suggestions

	CARBO-HYDRATES	PROTEIN	FAT	CALORIES
½ bagel with 1 tbsp grape or strawberry jam	45g	3g to 4g	0g	200
PB + honey sandwich: 2 slices low-fiber bread 1 tbsp peanut butter 2 tsp honey	40g	7g	3g	200
Low-fiber granola bar	30g to 60g	0g to 10g	0g to 5g	100 to 200

WHAT TO DRINK DURING EXERCISE

What you need to drink during exercise will depend on what your fueling choices are. Since the three main components an athlete needs to focus on during a competition are carbohydrates, electrolytes, and fluids, a drink choice should contain either one or all of these. As discussed previously, if you're someone who does well consuming a food-based fuel during exercise then your drink doesn't need to contain carbohydrates. In this case, the main focus should be on getting adequate fluids in, and potentially on supplementing electrolytes if your food doesn't contain sodium and potassium. For fluid needs alone, you should aim to consume about four ounces of fluid every 15 minutes. To be realistic, though, it's unlikely that you will have the time to measure out your fluids. At best, you'll have a water bottle or your drink strategically placed on the sidelines for when you have a few spare seconds to grab it. For this reason, a better way to measure out your fluids during exercise is to think of each gulp of water as about 1 fluid ounce. This means that when you grab that bottle, you should aim for three to four big gulps every 15 minutes.

If you want to consume fluids without extra electrolytes or carbohydrates, water alone will meet your needs. If you find yourself struggling to get in enough water because it isn't palatable enough during your exercise, add in a very small amount of fruit juice.

If your goal is to consume fluid *and* electrolytes, there are many different beverage choices that don't contain extra carbohydrates. Many popular products on the market have zero-sugar or no-calorie versions of their normal formulas. In most cases, this means you'll be able to easily find a product that meets just your fluid and electrolyte needs. Also, a number of different water brands on the market have added electrolytes. There are pros and cons to each product, however. Zero-sugar or zero-calorie sports drinks are often flavored, which may promote increased fluid consumption, but are likely to contain artificial sweeteners or ingredients. Water with electrolytes is typically all-natural, but is often plain. The best choice is one that helps you stay hydrated easily and meet your goals.

If your goal is to consume fluids, electrolytes, *and* quick-digesting carbohydrates in your drink during exercise, a regular sports drink will do the job. As discussed previously in the hydration section of this book (page 22), most sports drinks on the market have already been formulated with quick-digesting carbohydrates (often with both glucose and fructose), electrolytes, and fluids in the right ratios. Consuming four ounces of a sports drink every 15 minutes will help you meet all of your hydration and fueling needs at the same time. You can either buy a product already on the market for ease, or make your own if you want to go a more natural route (page 157).

Mid-Exercise Fluid Suggestions (Pick One)*

	CARBO-HYDRATES	PROTEIN	FAT	CALORIES	CONTAINS ELECTRO-LYTES
16 fl oz sports drink	40g	0g	0g	160	Yes
2 energy gels + 32 fl oz waterr	50g	0g	0g	200	Yes
16 fl oz sugar-free/ zero-calorie sports drink	0g	0g	0g	0	Yes
16 fl oz electrolyte water	0g	0g	0g	0	Yes
16 fl oz water	0g	0g	0g	0	No

For liquid fuel choices, it is recommended that you consume 4 fluid ounces every 15 minutes.

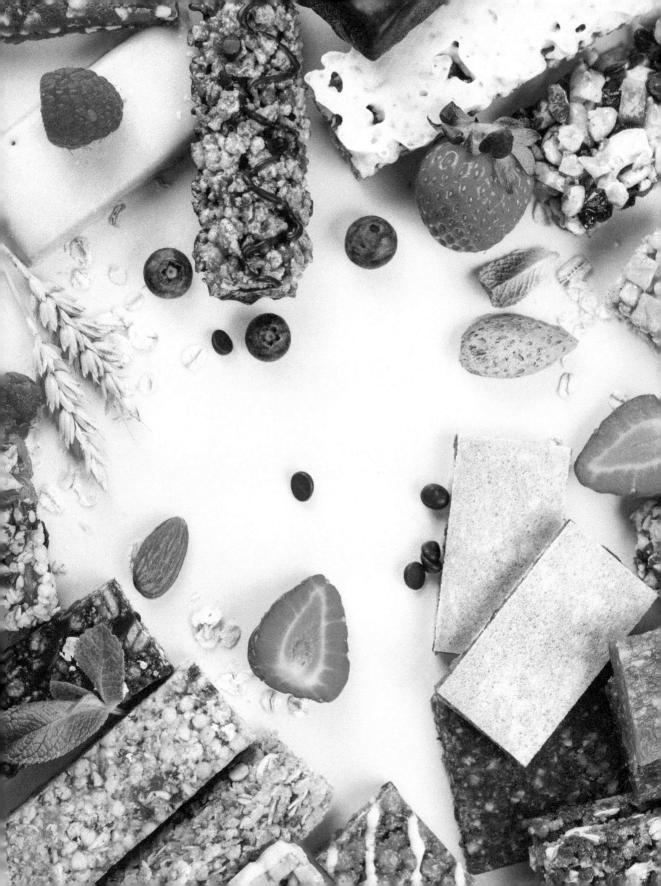

CHAPTER FIVE

POST-EXERCISE AND REST DAY FUEL

ONE OF THE MOST COMMON QUESTIONS I receive as a sports dietitian is, "What should an athlete eat after a training session or competition to refuel?" Choosing the right foods post-exercise allows the body to adequately recover its energy stores, provides nutrients to rebuild muscles, and gets the body those needed vitamins and minerals in order to maintain proper equilibrium.

WHAT TO EAT POST-EXERCISE

If you were to ask most people what they think the most important nutrient is to consume after exercise, you'd likely get protein as an answer. Most young adults think of protein when they think of a post-exercise fuel source, because protein is necessary to help rebuild muscles after a workout or exercise session. And while this is true, protein is actually not the most important nutrient that an athlete should be focusing on.

After a long training session or game, whether it be endurance-focused or strength-focused, your body has likely been depleted of glycogen, which needs to be quickly restored. Many studies suggest that the quicker glycogen is replenished after a training session, the faster an athlete will recover and the less likely he or she is to suffer from post-workout-related fatigue. For this reason, it is recommended to get a post-exercise fuel source within 30 to 60 minutes of finishing your exercise.

The main goal of the post-exercise meal is to replenish glycogen stores with quick-digesting carbohydrates, while also providing some protein to aid in muscle recovery. As a rule of thumb, you want to consume a 4:1 ratio of carbohydrates to protein in a post-exercise fuel source. You also want to get in a minimum of 40 grams of carbohydrates. So, as a minimum, using the 4:1 rule, a post-workout fuel should include roughly 40 grams of carbohydrates and 10 grams of protein.

MEALS VS. SNACKS

In a perfect world, you would get in a full post-exercise meal with the right ratio of carbohydrates to protein to meet an athlete's needs. But that's not always feasible for an athlete. Between putting equipment away, time in the locker room, and the commute home, it's unlikely that most young adults will be able to get a full meal in directly after exercise. In this case, it's recommended that you have a smaller post-exercise snack using the 4:1 guideline followed by a full recovery meal within two to three hours after exercising.

Post-Exercise Snack Suggestions

	CARBOHYDRATES	PROTEIN	CALORIES
16 fl oz low-fat chocolate milk	40g	11g	200
½ sandwich: 1 slice bread 2 oz low-sodium deli meat (ham, turkey, chicken) + 1 large apple	40g	14g	240
½ tuna pouch (1.5 oz) + 12 saltine crackers	30g	11g	145
2 low-fat cheese sticks + 1 oz pretzels + ½ banana	40g	14g	240

WHAT TO DRINK POST-EXERCISE

The goal of post-exercise fluid consumption is to ensure that an athlete gets enough fluids to replace what has been lost from training. Since every athlete will sweat and lose fluids differently based on their own unique physiology and training intensity, the best way to determine post-exercise fluid needs is to calculate them based on your own unique water loss.

To calculate how much fluid you should be consuming post-exercise:

1. Weigh yourself immediately before practice. This is your pre-exercise or natural weight before activity.

2. Weigh yourself immediately after practice. This is your post-exercise weight.

3. Calculate the difference. If you weighed 150 pounds before your practice and 147 pounds immediately after practice, then your body lost approximately 3 pounds of weight during that time. This weight difference is the amount of fluid lost in practice.

4. For every pound of water lost, aim to replace it immediately after practice with 16 to 24 fluid ounces (two to two and a half cups) of water. For example, if you lost three pounds of water weight during practice, your rehydration goal range would be:

- 16 fluid ounces x 3 pounds = 48 fluid ounces to
- 24 fluid ounces x 3 pounds = 72 fluid ounces

Tip: Depending on the type of workout or seasonality of your sport, your training intensity can vary greatly from one month to the next. As a minimum, it's recommended that you retest your fluid losses during practice every time there is a change in your training regimen (i.e., pre-season workouts, in-season workouts, post-season workouts) to get a ballpark of how your fluid needs should adjust. Additionally, the time of the year can also play a role in how much fluid you need, depending on whether your practice is indoors, outdoors, or in extreme heat or cold.

WHAT TO EAT ON REST DAY

Think of eating on a rest day as recharging your phone after a long day of use. Your battery is low, and you need to provide your body with the proper nutrients so that it can get back up to 100 percent power. Rest days are days when you have no formal exercise. In other words, a rest day can be one where you have small bouts of naturally planned physical activity such as walking or being active in normal day-to-day activities, but not one where there is a practice or a training regimen scheduled. If your day does include some kind of planned exercise, please use the guidelines in the pre-exercise, during exercise, and post-exercise sections of this chapter to come up with an adequate fueling plan.

Luckily, what a young adult needs on rest day doesn't differ greatly from what they need on a normal basis. Rest day nutrition should focus on having balanced meals that contain a mixture of complex carbohydrates (whole grains or whole wheat, vegetables, and fruit), protein, and healthy fat sources. While you do want to ensure adequate carbohydrate intake during rest in order to continue to restore glycogen stores, your specific needs aren't necessarily higher, so aiming for the recommended ranges of carbohydrates, protein, and fat that were calculated in chapter 1 (page 5) will suffice. As we discussed previously, having a balance of different macro- and micronutrients on the plate will ensure a varied and beneficial number of vitamins, minerals, and nutrients necessary to fuel the body for recovery.

Tip: Many athletes are concerned about consuming too many calories on rest days since their physical activity and, therefore, calorie needs will be lower compared to days when they are exerting themselves. One common pitfall is for athletes to try to recalculate their calorie and macronutrient needs and then be following two different plans, depending on which days they have planned exercise or not. A much simpler way to go about this is to just omit any exercise-related meals or snacks from your day. By simply not consuming your pre-exercise and post-exercise meal or snack, you'll be hitting your lower energy requirements without worry.

WHAT TO DRINK ON REST DAY

Just like proper food, fluids cannot be ignored simply because there is no planned exercise on a rest day. As with training days, adequate fluids are still necessary to maintain energy levels and proper body functioning. Fluids are necessary for the transport of certain vitamins and minerals, and as such, the body requires adequate fluid to recover properly. There are several ways to calculate your baseline fluid needs or rest day fluid requirements. One of the simplest is to take your current weight in pounds and divide it by two to get an estimate of your baseline hydration needs without having to take into account any additional exercise. So, if you're 150 pounds, then your baseline needs would be roughly 75 fluid ounces per day.

The body can only process a certain amount of water at a time, so don't try to front-load your daily water intake. Instead, space out your water consumption throughout the day. If you're awake for 16 hours a day, divide your total daily baseline needs by 16 to get a better idea of how many ounces of water to aim for each hour.

PART III

Personalized Needs of Individual Athletes

THERE IS NO ONE-SIZE-FITS-ALL when it comes to a performance nutrition plan. All athletes need a unique plan based not only on themselves as individuals, but also on their specific sport type and level of play. A female swimmer will have dramatically different needs from a power athlete such as a bodybuilder or wrestler. Likewise, two male baseball players could have entirely different nutrition needs based on their ages, body composition, genetics, and personal goals for their sport. To determine your own unique needs and what type of plan to use, it's important to evaluate your individual needs based on your gender, biology, body composition goals, and unique sport in order to determine what specifically you should be fueling with. Luckily, there are a few simple guidelines you can follow to come up with an individualized plan that works best for you.

CHAPTER SIX

FACTORS THAT INFLUENCE NUTRITION NEEDS

COMING UP WITH THE IDEAL PLAN FOR AN ATHLETE is sort of like opening a combination lock. You can't just get *most* of the numbers correct and hope that it's going to open. The same can be said for a fueling strategy. You can create the most amazing performance plan in the world, but if it's not tailored to you personally, then you're not going to get the competitive edge you're looking for. Remember, being at peak performance means creating a plan that addresses the individual just as much as it does their training requirements. Because there are distinct differences among all athletes, a number of factors need to be taken into consideration for an individual athlete to be at peak performance.

GENDER

From a biological standpoint, there are many differences in male and female bodies and how these relate to athletic performance. These changes aren't as noticeable with young athletes, but they do come into play upon hitting puberty. For women, this change coincides with increases in estrogen and up to a 33 percent increase in body fat during maturation. While this change is completely normal and healthy, some women can struggle with self-esteem and body image issues during the transition. For men, it is typically the opposite, as an increase in testosterone leads to increases in lean body mass and decreases in body fat. Additionally, most men develop a greater number of type 2 muscle fibers. These are muscle fibers related to generating large amounts of strength and speed compared to type 1 fibers, which are more geared toward muscular endurance. Testosterone also increases the number of red blood cells, which also helps male athletes have a greater endurance capacity. Both genders may develop mood swings, acne, and increased irritability during puberty. Regardless, all athletes are capable of greatness. A strong training, nutrition, and recovery plan can help overcome any obstacle and help athletes become champions. Female athletes need to ensure they're taking in enough energy or they risk irregular menstrual periods, loss of bone mineral density, and low energy availability. Further, weight-class sports, like wrestling, require extra care for women as water retention and weight are affected not only by food and fluids, but also by hormonal shifts during the month. Male athletes, on the other hand, are likely to have challenges related to body composition after puberty, including mood swings and higher energy demands.

WOMEN

Female athletes have a few unique challenges when entering puberty. In addition to changes in body composition and fat mass, women also have an increase in estrogen production during menstruation. This means female athletes may have challenges such as mood swings and changes in energy levels during their periods. Additionally, women are more prone to specific types of injuries, including shoulder injuries, knee injuries, and stress fractures. The good news is that by adequately planning ahead and having a solid warm-up, training, and cool-down regimen as well as planning proper nutrition, you can greatly reduce some of the negative side effects.

MEN

Male athletes also have some unique challenges. Once a young male athlete hits puberty, his body tends to produce a large amount of testosterone, which changes body composition. Male athletes tend to have a decrease in body fat and an increase in lean muscle mass as a result. The changes in hormones and body composition also bring about growth spurts, which can be particularly challenging for those who participate in weight-class sports. For instance, a one-inch increase in height is typically accompanied by several pounds of weight gain. While this is a normal part of growth, it can be frustrating for those who have to stay within a certain weight range for their sport. Puberty and hormonal shifts are also frequently accompanied by mood swings, irritability, sadness, or generalized frustration. Additionally, there are specific injury types that are more common in men. These include groin pulls, hamstring injuries, and ACL tears. Following a proper warm up, training, and cool down regimen along with proper nutrition can help minimize the risk of these injuries.

Men who are fully matured also have other obstacles to overcome. While body image disorders are most frequently talked about among women, they affect men as well. Not fitting into a certain body composition type or athletic *look* can create feelings of self-consciousness and inadequacy.

AGE

Age plays just as big a role in your nutritional needs as how active you are. Growth requires extremely large amounts of energy and nutrients to happen effectively. Picture growth like trying to build a house. You can make an amazing blueprint for a mansion, but if you're missing the materials to put your walls up and build a roof, your mansion likely won't come to fruition. Nutrition is the same way. When a body undergoes growth, which typically happens until roughly the age of 16 to 18, it requires a significantly higher number of calories and nutrient needs compared to someone whose body is no longer trying to generate new tissues, bone, or ligaments. Furthermore, age plays an interesting role in how the body stores certain nutrients. Some micronutrients, such as calcium, can only be stored at optimal levels when we're growing. How we store this mineral is similar to how we would put money into a savings account. At a younger age, you're able to deposit calcium regularly to keep it safe for the future. Once you reach the age of 19 or 20, however, you're no longer able to store any more calcium. This is because your body is now using or "withdrawing" roughly the same amount of calcium from your bones as it's able to deposit. Once you hit the age of 29 or 30, the calcium your body needs is taken directly out of that "savings account." If you didn't do a good job of saving when you were younger, you may run into issues later down the road when you need to make withdrawals. This is why it's extremely important to not only fuel your body calorie-wise for growth at a young age, but also to make sure you're getting a balanced variety of foods that have all of the macro- and micronutrients needed to sustain optimal health and performance both now and in the future.

BODY TYPE

Athletes can have almost as many different body types as there are different sports. There are a lot of sports nutrition supplement commercials showing athletes with six- and eight-pack abs, hulking amounts of muscle mass, and virtually no body fat, so it can be easy for you to think that this is what you're supposed to look like. The reality is that most athletes do not fit into this stereotype. While an active person may have more muscle mass than the average individual, athletes still commonly have many different body shapes. Some individuals are prone to storing their body fat in their midsection while having a leaner lower body. Others may have a relatively lean torso and more powerful leg muscles. Some women or men may be very curvy, while others have a straighter, leaner body type. No matter how much you work out, it isn't very feasible to change your type of body or to lose fat from a particular body part. Nor should you need to. All bodies can be capable of athleticism regardless of physical appearance.

An athlete or active young adult may also have issues surrounding overall weight if a health care provider is not aware of the differences in body composition between an average person and an athlete. For example, many strength athletes or those who have large amounts of muscle mass get their body mass index (BMI) checked by a health professional. BMI is a method of calculating whether an average person is considered underweight, within a healthy weight range, or overweight or obese. The point of checking BMI is not to shame an individual, but rather to get a rough idea of overall health status. Unfortunately, using BMI as a health indicator has many flaws, especially for athletes. Active individuals may fall into the category of overweight or even obese even though they're within a perfectly healthy weight range. The reason this happens is because the formula designed to assess an individual's health based on their weight and height alone does not take into account lean muscle mass. BMI will always be an inaccurate indicator of an athlete's health because lean mass is denser than fat mass, meaning an athlete may weigh more naturally even though muscle mass is a healthy type of lean tissue. BMI automatically assumes that all weight above a certain point is body fat, and therefore pushes the individual out of a *healthy* weight range.

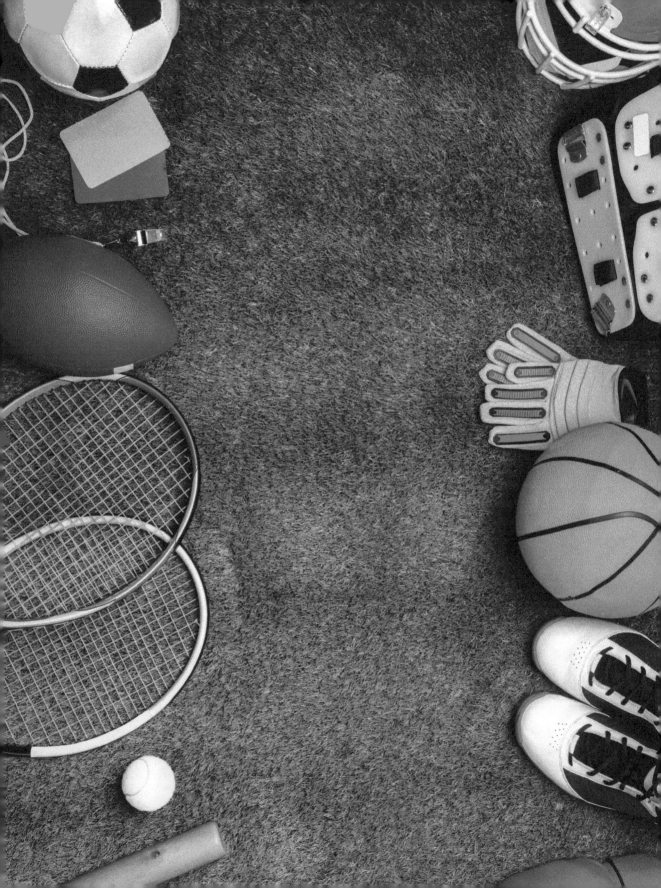

CHAPTER SEVEN

NUTRITION NEEDS BASED ON SPORT TYPE

TRUE OR FALSE: All sports have a similar level of training intensity, so the nutrient needs of athletes across different sports will be the same.

If you answered "false," you're correct. All sports have different challenges and priorities that require either small or large modifications in a performance plan to see success. An ultra-marathon runner has a dramatically different fueling goal from a power lifter, because the goals of their sports are entirely different. An active adult playing a team sport likely needs to focus on a combination of endurance and power output, while a long-distance runner may need to carefully plan out his or her fueling and hydration strategy to ensure their glycogen stores will last through an entire race. In this chapter, we're going to take a look at team sports, individual sports, and endurance training to show athletes what to focus on for their in-season and off-season goals.

TEAM SPORTS

Athletes in team sports are in a unique position of needing to be balanced in all areas of performance: strength, endurance, and agility. While every single sport, and even every position, may have a different role or focus, the majority of team athletes need to be well rounded in order to compete at their best. Just like your training needs to be diverse, nutrition must be well rounded as well. By focusing on a balanced plan throughout the season that covers all phases of training, you can ensure that you're eating and drinking the right foods and fluids to promote recovery, reduce inflammation, increase strength, and maintain your energy levels to outlast your opponents on the field or court.

BASEBALL AND SOFTBALL

Baseball and softball players have extremely demanding schedules, often playing 40 or even 50-plus games throughout the season. If your goal is to change your body composition by losing body fat, increasing muscle mass, or a combination of both, the off-season is the best time to make these changes. During the pre-season, establish a realistic performance nutrition plan. Look at your class schedule and training times to come up with an achievable plan. When in season, the main focus should be on optimizing performance during games and reducing recovery time as much as possible. Focus on carbohydrate-rich fuel sources around training times and competition. Additionally, if games include a lot of sprinting or are in extreme weather temperatures, it is especially important to follow a hydration plan to avoid fatigue. Follow our pre-workout nutrition guidelines in chapter 3 (page 39) and spread your meals out evenly throughout the day—instead of back-loading your calories after practice—to keep your body fueled and recovery time short.

One common pitfall for baseball and softball players is overestimating calorie needs. During low-intensity training sessions or off-days, carbohydrate requirements will be significantly lower than other team sports that have a more intense cardio component. Focus on whole-grain carbohydrate sources and be mindful of portion sizes during low-activity days to help balance out your calorie needs. Whole-grain carbohydrate sources include vegetables, fruits, beans, oatmeal, and brown or black rice. Additionally, know when to select water versus a sports drink. If your practice or game isn't in intense weather conditions (extreme hot or cold) or you're not consistently undergoing moderate physical activity for an hour or more, a sports drink likely isn't necessary.

BASKETBALL

Basketball players have the challenge of combining physical performance, mental toughness, and a large amount of technique and technical skill to achieve greatness. Your fueling needs will vary depending on what phase of training you're in. For the pre-season, focus on creating a realistic performance plan that takes into account your schedule and practice times. Since basketball players have been known to run several miles in any given practice or game, it's important to focus on pre- and post-workout snacks and meals to keep energy and glycogen levels up (refer to part II, pages. 39–43, for specific snack and meal examples). For games, aim to eat a pre-competition meal that is rich in carbohydrates around 3 to 4 hours before tip-off. During time-outs, bench time, or other breaks during games, refuel with either a quick-digesting carbohydrate source or liquid fuel in addition to replenishing liquids. Depending on your play time and sweat rate, an electrolyte beverage maybe better than plain water.

FOOTBALL

Football players come in a variety of shapes and sizes, and a particular athlete's position on the field is often size dependent as much as it is skill dependent. Like most sports, the best time to set goals for changing body composition is in the off-season, typically beginning for most in June or July. This will give you ample time to make steady changes and reach your goals before ramping up for the season. If you're struggling to keep weight on, focus on adding energy-dense calories to your nutrition plan, such as nuts, nut butters, seeds, cheeses, avocado, or guacamole. If you're looking to lose body fat, focus on filling your plate with lean proteins (chicken, fish, or turkey), colorful fruits and vegetables, and whole-grain sources of carbohydrates. During the pre-season, establish your nutrition and hydration plan based on your class and training schedules.

Depending on equipment and weather conditions, football players can sweat at a much higher rate than those in other team sports. Choosing an electrolyte beverage instead of plain water will help replenish fluids and keep you hydrated. In-season games require a fueling focus that maximizes a lot of short, intense bursts of physical activity. During a timeout, halftime, or other breaks, it is imperative that you refuel with quick-digesting carbohydrates. Since football is also a contact sport, you may tolerate liquid fuel better than food-based carbohydrates, as they are digested very quickly.

HOCKEY

Hockey players have games that are three periods in length, with each period lasting approximately 20 minutes. While substitutions are common, and players are rarely on the ice the entire time, the game itself requires periods of very intense activity. Therefore, athletes should focus on building strength and working on body composition in the off-season. Since hockey players often sweat heavily due to a combination of the competition intensity and their gear, a proper fluid plan is a must. Time your fluid intake around your substitutions and breaks. Further, be sure to include electrolytes and quick-digesting carbohydrates in your fluids if your practice is greater than one hour or you are unable to tolerate solid fuel. Since game breaks are short, it may be necessary to periodically refuel a small amount at every break instead of trying to fit in your fluids and/or food at one time. Too much food or fluid in one sitting may cause cramping or GI distress, especially during this contact sport. After competitions, a hockey player's priority should be refueling glycogen with quick-digesting carbohydrates such as fruits, low-fiber granola bars, or a sandwich on white bread. Incorporating a small amount of protein to repair muscle tissues is ideal. Aim for lean protein sources such as turkey, chicken, or fish.

LACROSSE

Lacrosse players require a complex skill set to be victorious, including constantly switching between low-intensity and high-intensity activity when it comes to game time. Because lacrosse is such a demanding sport, it is not uncommon for athletes to skip meals or forget to hydrate throughout the days or weeks leading up to a competition. Lacrosse players should emphasize daily nutrition plans that focus on performance fueling in order to avoid fatigue, cramps, and potential injury. Aim for balanced meals in the pre-season to properly fuel the body with carbohydrates, protein, and fat. Additionally, the pre-season is the time to determine your class schedule and upcoming training schedule in order to plot out when you'll have fueling and hydration breaks throughout the day. If your goal is to put on weight or if you struggle to maintain your current weight, aim to include foods such as nuts, nut butters, tuna pouches, avocado, or legumes into your daily meals for a quick calorie boost. During game days, make sure you have a pregame and postgame fueling and hydration plan. Keep a bottle of water or sports drink on the sideline to take small sips of throughout the competition. Halftime will be a lacrosse player's main opportunity to refuel, so pack a quick-digesting carbohydrate source or additional sports drink to replenish fluids, glycogen, and electrolytes.

SOCCER

Soccer players may have one of the most intense endurance requirements out of any team sport. Many times, an athlete on the field will play the full 45 minutes of a game half without a substitution and with minimal rest time. For this reason, soccer players need to focus on strategically getting in both hydration and carbohydrates. The pre-season is when players should focus on making body composition changes, as you often have a more intense strength training regimen during this time. Since fueling needs aren't as high during the pre-season, limit your liquid calories and avoid having a pre- or post-workout nutrition snack on low-intensity or rest days. During the pre-season, set up your fueling plan based on your class and training schedules to help you keep on track during hectic days when the season begins. Ensure that your fueling plan is realistic based on when and how often you can eat throughout the day. During the season, your emphasis should be on promoting quick recovery between practices as well as staying properly hydrated and fueled during each half of a game. Getting a pre-workout snack or meal in as well as a post-workout fuel source consumed within 30 minutes of practice should be a priority. During games, it may not be possible to stop for fluids or food breaks every 15 minutes. If this is the case, be sure to pack an electrolyte beverage and a quick-digesting carbohydrate, such as low-fiber granola bars, bananas, or half of a turkey or chicken sandwich on low-fiber bread. If you're frequently hungry while on the field, pack extra servings of these foods to keep you pleasantly fueled and able to focus on the match.

VOLLEYBALL

Volleyball players not only have intense training demands, but are also required to maintain a very high amount of lean body mass to support the balance of strength, endurance, and power required during matches. Because volleyball is so dynamic, nutrition needs shift depending on the time of the season. Focus on building a strong base plan in the off-season that includes a diet rich in protein to support muscle mass growth during resistance training. After the season begins, it is important to map out exactly when classes and training times fall so that you can fit mini-meals or snacks in between. Volleyball practice and competition are often held at night, so a good goal is to spread your fueling plan out adequately throughout the day. If there is not enough time to have sufficient dinner 3 to 4 hours before a training session or game, plan to have a snack 2 to 3 hours prior that is rich in carbohydrates with a small amount of protein and fat. An hour before competition or training, have a carbohydrate-based snack that is low in fiber, such as a banana or sports drink, to top off your glycogen levels, and then have a complete dinner meal after practice. Like many other team sports, you may not have more than a few moments for a break in between games, so it's advisable to keep a sports drink within reach to take a few gulps periodically throughout a match.

ENDURANCE SPORTS

Endurance athletes are in the unique position of requiring a constant flow of glycogen during prolonged activity to fuel muscles. Unlike athletes participating in traditional sports, endurance athletes must carefully match their carbohydrate intake to their training intensity or else they're likely to "bonk" or "hit the wall." In addition to adequate carbohydrate intake, it is also imperative that athletes have enough protein to maintain their current lean body mass. Without this, endurance athletes may become weaker throughout the season. Decreased carbohydrate intake can also lead to issues like cramping, nausea, or even vomiting if an adequate fuel plan is not in place.

CYCLING

Cyclists require a combination of endurance and optimal power output to get ahead of the competition. Much like athletes in other endurance sports, cyclists need to focus on topping off glycogen stores by having adequate carbohydrates before, during, and after competition. In order to maintain energy levels throughout long races, you need 30 to 60 grams of quick-digesting carbohydrates, electrolytes, and an additional 16 to 32 fluid ounces of water for every hour of riding. Additionally, you need to be mindful of your body composition. The goal of most cyclists is to be as lean as possible while still maintaining adequate power output. For this reason, you should pay special attention to ensuring you're getting adequate protein to maintain lean body mass. If your goal is to reduce body fat and overall size, then you should follow a very gradual weight loss plan of 0.5 to 1 pound per week. By doing so, you will avoid dramatic losses in strength during the process.

MARATHON RUNNING

Marathons can range anywhere from a little over 26 miles for a full marathon to 13 miles for a half marathon. One of the most common pre-marathon rituals that athletes partake in is carbohydrate loading the night before a race. The goal is to increase the amount of glycogen that the body can hold. A good rule of thumb for carbohydrate loading is to consume roughly 70 percent of your total calories from carbohydrates. But, like all other aspects of performance nutrition, carbohydrate loading is very individualized and will affect each athlete differently. Some marathoners may see and feel a difference in their endurance and running times, while others won't. Just like running in general, the priority for marathoners on race day is to ensure you're getting adequate glycogen, electrolytes, and fluids every hour throughout the event. Like most runners, marathoners should consume 30 to 60 grams of quick-digesting carbohydrates, electrolytes, and 4 to 8 fluid ounces of water for every 15 minutes you're hitting the dirt or pavement. Unlike cross country running, however, a runner's belt is likely not going to hold enough to meet a marathoner's fuel or fluid needs. For this reason, it is important for you to pace your refueling properly and take advantage of any rest and hydration stations along the way. Most races will have booths set up along the course, and while it may seem smart to skip these in favor of reducing your finish time, you still need to properly recharge along the way. Equipment such as a hydration pack may be a better alternative, so runners can avoid pit stops. While some marathon runners can tolerate small amounts of solid foods, such as half of a banana or a handful of pretzels, most get GI distress when trying to eat during a run. For this reason, sticking with liquid fuel choices may be a better alternative.

RUNNING AND CROSS COUNTRY

In general, runners need to ensure that they're consistently and adequately replacing glycogen stores for any run or activity lasting an hour or longer. Running poses a few unique challenges, though. Most runners simply do not have the ability to stop for a food or snack break in the middle of activity, so your only options are liquid fuel sources or easily consumable carbohydrates like gels. The main fueling focus for a runner should be to ensure adequate fluid, electrolyte, and carbohydrate intake. In general, runners should be replacing their glycogen stores with 30 to 60 grams of quick-digesting carbohydrates every hour. The amount of fluid you need will vary, but a good place to start is 4 to 8 fluid ounces for every 15 minutes of exercise. One of the biggest obstacles for runners is not having a fluid and fueling source on hand, since bottles can be bulky and irritating to hold during runs. For those who have trouble with this, investing in a runner's belt with water pouch slots can help. If that isn't possible, be sure to drink 8 to 16 fluid ounces of water within half an hour of beginning a run and replace every pound of water weight lost with 16 to 24 fluid ounces of a sports drink after.

SWIMMING

Swimmers have some of the most intense training regimens of any endurance athlete at the high school and collegiate level. With a mix of swim practice and field practice, swim athletes are trained to balance their power output with their speed and energy levels in order to hit their time splits. During the off-season, a swimmer's energy needs are significantly lower than when actively engaging in the sport. Be sure to taper down your energy intake as your training regimen slows down by removing your pre- and post-activity fuel from your nutrition plan. If your goal is body composition changes to improve performance, the off-season is also the time to plan this, as the body won't suffer as much from a lower energy intake. During the season, you will need to ensure that you are getting adequate carbohydrates and hydration around practice and competition times. A common mistake swimmers make is to not take the time to hydrate, either because they don't recognize thirst in the first place, or because they lack the time to do so while in the pool. Since there is likely little time to stop for a hydration break, let alone eat a snack, you will have to get creative to get fuel. Leaving a sports drink at one or both ends of the pool while doing laps can help you sneak a few gulps in throughout practice. This will help keep your body fueled throughout and ensure proper hydration. After practice and competition, the focus should be on getting quick-digesting carbohydrates into the body to further top off glycogen stores. You should also ingest 15 to 20 grams of protein to help repair muscle tissue.

STRENGTH TRAINING SPORTS

Strength-based sports often rely on strategically timed fueling and resistance training to help meet power output and muscle mass goals. Most strength-related sports are not only about improving power output, but are also centered on a specific type of physique goal or weight class. Because of this, it is extremely important for most strength athletes to ensure they are getting adequate calories and are strategically creating a fueling plan based on what season they are in and their body composition goals. Unlike endurance athletes, strength-related sports typically require less caloric intake due to the stop-and-go intensity of the sports. A proper performance plan can help strength athletes determine what their focus should be on (body composition goals versus performance) and create a year-long plan to reach those goals successfully. One pitfall for most strength athletes is knowing exactly when to modify body composition. Because it is extremely difficult for the body to gain muscle mass while at a caloric deficit, most athletes will have to break their nutrition regimen down into a "cutting" phase where they lose body fat and a "bulking" phase if their goal is to gain muscle mass.

BODYBUILDING

Bodybuilders aren't your typical gym-goers who enjoy lifting weights on occasion. These athletes often do some form of resistance training for two to three hours at a time, most days of the week. The goal of most bodybuilders is to build as much lean mass as possible while keeping body fat down. Many will often even compete on stage in bikini, fitness, or physique competitions where they are judged based on their physical appearance and body composition. Bodybuilders in particular must cycle through different performance plans during the year depending on their goals. Since it is extremely difficult to build muscle mass and lose body fat at the same time because the body is in a caloric deficit, it is often necessary to break these two goals down into separate plans. For instance, you may spend a handful of months out of the year where you are "bulking" to build up lean body mass. In these cases, a gradual weight gain of 0.5 to 1 pound per week is advisable. While some may think bulking means to put on as much weight as possible, the goal is not to put on any type of weight, but specifically lean mass. While the rate of lean mass an individual is able to put on varies based on their training history, current regimen, and diet, it should still be done in a very controlled and gradual way to get the best results. Simply adding 250 to 500 calories to your daily nutrition plan should be enough to spur muscle growth. A pre-lifting meal that is rich in carbohydrates with a moderate amount of protein, as well as a post-lifting snack with 20 grams of protein and 45 to 60 grams of carbohydrates, is a good place to start to ensure proper recovery and growth. Likewise, when "cutting" weight, you want to aim for no more than a 250- to 500-calorie deficit per week to avoid losing muscle mass as much as possible. Because the body is in a caloric deficit, it may be necessary to increase protein intake slightly to preserve lean muscle mass.

CROSSFIT

CrossFit athletes range from general workout enthusiasts who enjoy going to a box to get their scheduled activity in, all way to elite athletes who compete at national-level competitions. Because of this, nutrition needs will vary from one individual to the next. The goal of most general workout enthusiasts is to "get in shape" and possibly make some gains on their lifts. For this population, given that a typical CrossFit workout is only 60 minutes from start to end (including warm-ups and cool-downs), an intense performance plan may not be necessary. Rather, these individuals should simply focus on balanced meals throughout the day. If necessary, they should also ensure that they are getting carbohydrates prior to their workout and a carbohydrate and protein source within 30 minutes of completing their workout to help repair muscle tissue and recover properly before their next scheduled class. In contrast, elite athletes who do CrossFit often train more than 60 minutes per day and will include various other forms of activity outside of their traditional Workout of the Day (WOD). These athletes in particular should pay closer attention to their fueling plan to ensure they're adequately matching their caloric intake to their energy expenditure and getting in the proper pre- and post-workout meals or snacks. As a rule of thumb, aim for 45 to 60 grams of carbohydrates and 15 to 20 grams of protein after an intense workout to aid recovery.

WRESTLING

Wrestling is a unique sport in that athletes must adhere to specific weight classes during most tournaments. These weight classes have a weigh-in portion and may require wrestlers to meet their weight requirements the night before or half an hour before the start of a match. This means that wrestlers must constantly maintain their weight throughout the season to avoid being taken out of the lineup. And while younger athletes (middle school or lower) may have the option to bump up or down a class to suit their growing bodies, high school and collegiate level athletes are often locked into their class. One of the most important things you can do is follow proper weight management nutrition throughout the entire season. Even then, incidents like growth spurts or limited weight class selection can cause wrestlers to compete in a class above or below their "natural" weight. For a wrestler, focusing on weight maintenance throughout the year and a diet that is nutrient-dense with particular attention to pre- and post-training fuel sources will have a big impact on your performance on the mat. For those who are sitting above their weight class naturally and need to *make weight* for a competition, choosing very low-sodium and unprocessed foods while focusing on hydration in the days leading up to a weigh-in will help prevent the body from retaining extra fluids.

OTHER COMPETITIVE SPORTS

While many sports fit easily into categories such as team, strength, and endurance-driven, others require a different level of athleticism or mental acuity. Because these sports have unique training demands and nutritional requirements, they've been put into their own separate category and will be covered here.

GOLF

The skill and competitiveness of golfers can vary from a general enthusiast who likes getting on the green once or twice a week to those competing at an elite level at national or even international tournaments. Therefore, the nutritional needs of golfers will also vary. In general, golf is a game primarily determined by skill, but there are still some physical demands to the sport. Most golfers will be on the green for three to five hours playing an 18-hole game, and for those who are serious athletes, this may be followed by a training session that could be strength-based, endurance-based, or a combination of the two. In addition, golfers could walk anywhere from four to eight miles or more during a game. For this reason, you should be sure that you get a balanced and adequate meal in prior to stepping onto the green. Having a meal rich in carbohydrates with moderate amounts of protein and fat will help keep you energized and satiated throughout. Additionally, hydration needs to be a component for any golfer's performance plan. Dehydration not only can cause physical symptoms, but can also affect the mental side of the sport by causing brain fog or issues with focusing. Severe dehydration can make a golfer prone to heat stroke, if the weather during play time is considered extreme. While a sports drink may not be necessary, you should bring adequate water onto the course and ensure that you are drinking regularly.

GYMNASTICS

While most think of gymnastics as a completely endurance-related sport, gymnasts are constantly undergoing a breakdown of muscle and connective tissue during their practices, particularly in landings. Because of this, gymnasts constantly need to ensure adequate carbohydrate and protein intake, as the body is always recovering and repairing. Gymnastics gets complicated further by the fact that most athletes are looking to maintain a specific body composition or size in an attempt to better their routine or have an easier time maintaining a perfect form during competitions. Because of this, many gymnasts are caught between trying to fuel properly while purposely restricting energy consumption to get down to an "ideal size." While it is possible to get all of your nutrient needs from a balanced diet, gymnasts may want to supplement with a multivitamin that contains calcium and vitamin D. This will help ensure adequate nutrient intake as well as provide the body with additional fuel sources to build strong bones. Since gymnasts are prone to stress fracture, these supplements will help fight back.

The pre-season for a gymnast can be very strenuous, with many teams having two-a-day practices that last for several hours. During this time, you should focus on a carbohydrate-rich diet. On average, most gymnasts need approximately 5 to 7 grams of carbohydrates per kilogram of body weight during the pre-season. During the season, as training intensity winds down slightly, your carbohydrate needs will be reduced to approximately 4 to 6 grams of carbohydrates per kilogram of body weight. In the post-season, carbohydrate needs decline further as activity is reduced even more, and most gymnasts will only need 4 grams of carbohydrates per kilogram of body weight. When creating a nutrition plan, be sure to plan out when, where, and how long your meets are. Account for both travel time and activity when you create your schedule. If you'll be traveling long distances, it may be necessary to pack shelf-stable pre- and post-activity snacks or meals such as tuna pouches with crackers, fruits like bananas or apples, or low-fiber granola bars, in addition to adequate fluids. If you're exercising for an hour or greater at a moderate intensity, a sports drink with electrolytes may help top off energy stores and maintain proper hydration status. During the off-season, it's important for gymnasts to take a few weeks off to rest and recover adequately, as the body has been put under an enormous stress load during the season.

TENNIS

Balancing the needs to fuel for endurance as well as for short bursts of energy requires tennis athletes to have a balanced fueling plan all season long. Tennis players can often fall into a rut of being dehydrated and not properly fueled on the court when trying to balance work or school schedules with practice. Develop a fueling and hydration plan early on to address nutrition needs. In the pre-season, you should focus on consuming adequate fluids, having a balanced diet with fruits and vegetables, and following a proper recovery plan. During any training or competition, always have a water bottle or sports drink on hand. Since tennis is often played in extreme heat or humid conditions, athletes are especially prone to dehydration. Proper hydration throughout the entire day as well as during practice and games is essential to keep energy levels and concentration high and to avoid injuries. You should aim for 8 fluid ounces of water every 15 minutes during activity. After a practice or match, you should consume a meal or snack with a combination of carbohydrates and protein to aid in recovery.

TRACK (SHORT DISTANCE)

Short distance track runners (i.e., sprinters) have very unique nutritional focuses. A sprinter's main objective is to produce enough power and have the short bursts of energy required to hit his or her times. Because of this, carbohydrate loading isn't necessary. Instead, sprinters should focus on a diet that facilitates muscle mass growth when trying to improve lean mass, and focus on maintenance at all other times. Focusing on a combination of complex carbohydrates, protein, and fat at most meals will provide adequate energy for short-distance track athletes. If you find you're within an hour of a competition and you haven't recently had a fuel source, then a quick-digesting carbohydrate such as a banana or low-fiber granola bar can help top off your energy stores. Additionally, daily hydration will be key to avoiding fatigue or delayed reaction times during an event.

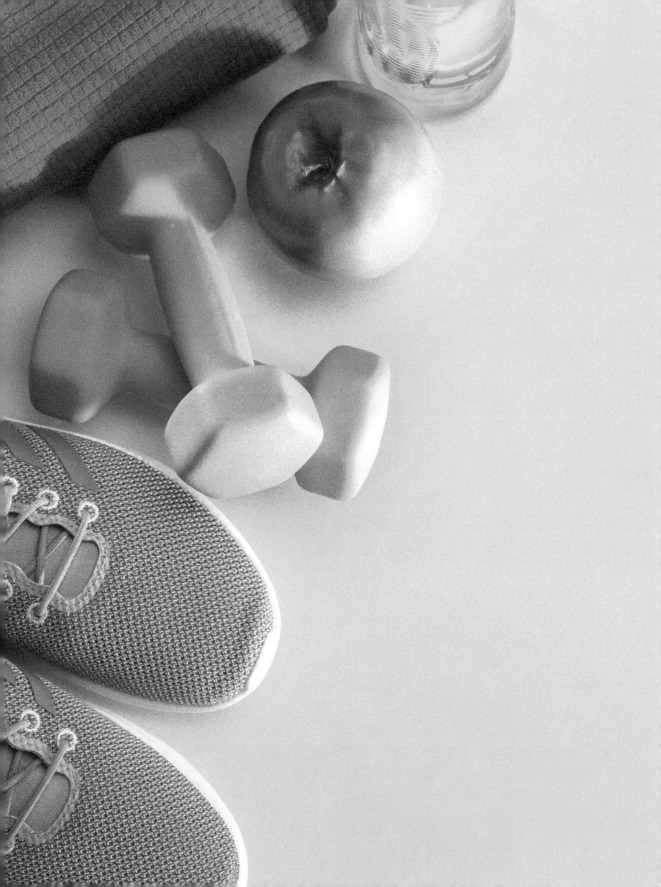

CHAPTER EIGHT

BALANCING WEIGHT AND NUTRITION

MANAGING WEIGHT AS AN ATHLETE can come naturally, or it can be one of the biggest challenges an active individual will face. Some athletes will struggle to keep weight on even if they feel like they're eating 24/7, while others may have trouble getting down to what they deem an appropriate weight for their sport. Regardless of where an athlete falls on this spectrum, there are a number of reasons or challenges that could cause an athlete to want to change his or her body weight. Some athletes may need to adhere to a specific weight class, which forces them to either increase or decrease their weight so that they can compete. Other athletes may be looking to lose weight to gain a greater power advantage in their sport, such as gymnasts, cyclists, and swimmers. Others still may simply be so active that they find it difficult to stay at a healthy and sustainable weight, because they burn so many calories on a daily basis and their hunger cues aren't matching up with their energy requirements. In situations like these, athletes should very strategically consider why and how they're looking to make body composition changes. Gaining or losing weight too quickly can actually have a negative effect on performance. When an athlete puts weight on too fast, he or she is likely putting on a significant amount of that weight as body fat. Likewise, when weight is lost too quickly, it's often done to the detriment of lean muscle mass and can affect the athlete's strength. For these reasons, a proper weight loss or gain plan needs to be constructed that considers the training needs of the athlete as well as where in the season he or she is.

Tip: Not all athletes are looking to change their weight for performance boosts. Many individuals may simply be looking to change their body weight or body composition because they're self-conscious about their appearance or are looking to fit in to a certain stereotype or crowd. It's important for athletes in these situations to know that what the media portrays as a typical athletic body is not the norm. It is completely normal for athletes to come in all shapes and sizes. Some athletes may be naturally thin while others are curvy. Some may hold fat in their mid-section while others hold it in their lower body. And cellulite is completely normal regardless of someone's body fat percentage. The next time you look in the mirror and worry about not matching a certain look, challenge yourself instead to name three amazing things your body does for you—whether that's being able to run several miles, go through hours of intense practice without failing, or lift double or even triple its own weight in times of stress. Every body is unique and strong in its own way.

WEIGHT LOSS

When individuals picture weight loss, they often think of skipping meals or tiny portion sizes that leave them hungry, fatigued, and just a bit miserable. As you can imagine, this is extremely counterproductive not only to general weight loss efforts, but also to athletic performance. Athletes need to lose weight at a very controlled and gradual pace. If they don't, they risk feeling fatigued throughout the day, which will affect their game or match. Moreover, they may lose a significant amount of weight from muscle mass (i.e., strength) versus body fat. When weight loss is too rapid, the body will pull energy from muscles to sustain itself. Luckily, there are a few things you can do to lose weight safely without risking your performance or strength:

1. Aim for a gradual weight loss of 0.5 to 1 pound per week if possible. A controlled weight descent goal can be met by simply reducing calorie needs by 250 to 500 per day. You can easily achieve this by replacing certain foods such as whole-fat milk or yogurts with their low-fat counterparts, and avoiding too many servings of energy-dense foods like fried foods, bakery items, nuts, and oil. Having a slow weight loss plan will allow you to continue competing without dramatically reducing your fuel sources and/or energy levels. It also allows you to ensure that you're holding on to as much of your muscle mass as possible and losing as much body fat as possible instead.

2. Don't cut out entire food groups. It's common for athletes to simply cut out starchy carbohydrates or other food groups as a simple way to reduce their caloric intake. This, however, can lead to a lack of nutrients and adequate energy coming to the body.

3. Don't overly restrict food choices. Just like cutting out entire food groups is unhealthy, it can also be counterproductive to try to eat clean 100 percent of the time. While you don't want to eat entire pizzas or order fast food on a regular basis, you do need balance when it comes to choosing foods you enjoy and those that provide fuel. Ironically, when athletes cut out processed foods completely, they often begin obsessing over the foods they *can't* eat and may end up binging on those same items later. Instead, having a plan that favors moderation and allows for some foods on occasion even though they're not the optimal choice will lead to better overall compliance.

4. Get adequate rest. Getting the right amount of sleep isn't just important for recovery and energy balance. Sleep deprivation has actually been shown to cause changes in hormones, particularly the hormones that affect hunger and satiety levels. Individuals who don't get adequate sleep are more likely to consume extra calories throughout the day compared to those who get seven to nine hours.

5. Set up your environment for success. It's a lot easier to stay on track with proper nutrition if your house or environment is filled with healthy choices. If a tray of brownies is on the counter instead, you'll likely reach for the treat. If you have a fruit bowl sitting on your kitchen counter instead, you'll be more likely to reach for an apple the next time you want a snack. Environment trumps an athlete's so-called willpower every time, so take extra steps to make sure the foods you want to eat are readily available.

6. Eat less on rest days. A common pitfall for athletes is to create a performance plan based on their training schedule and continue to follow that plan even on rest days or in the off-season. A simple way to modify a plan for success is to leave out any pre-exercise or post-exercise fueling choices. This will automatically reduce calories throughout the day without needing to completely change your plan.

7. Move more. An interesting phenomenon happens to active individuals: To compensate for increased activity during sports or training, some individuals may reduce the amount of movement or activity they do for the rest of the day without even realizing it. Make a conscious effort to continue moving, even if it isn't during a practice. Even small things like taking the stairs instead of an elevator or going on a walk with friends can make a difference over the course of a week in how active you are and how much energy you burn.

WEIGHT GAIN

Weight gain can be just as difficult for some individuals as weight loss. Given how active some athletes are, it can be very hard for them to eat enough calories to simply maintain weight, let alone gain. However, many times an athlete may need to gain weight. For example, a wrestler looking to compete in a specific weight class may need to put on a few pounds in order to get to where he or she needs to be. But just like with weight loss, proper weight gain needs to be done strategically and gradually. A common pitfall for many athletes is using weight gain as an excuse to eat a large amount of energy-dense foods, such as pizza, dessert, and fast food, under the guise of "bulking up." But ideal weight gain for an athlete should happen at a rate of 0.5 to 1 pound per week. Weight gain should be slow and steady to avoid putting on the wrong kind of weight. When weight gain is too quick, then the majority of the weight gained is in the form of body fat, which only hinders performance. Instead, a gradual weight gain while engaging in resistance training or exercise helps ensure that some of the weight being put on is in additional muscle mass instead of fat mass. Athletes also want to make sure they're still eating a proper diet for weight gain. Most often, this means consuming the same types of foods they were previously, just in bigger portion sizes. For athletes, the goal of putting on weight should be to compete better, not worse, because of their diet.

To better formulate a weight gain plan, athletes should plan in advance when they need to be at their goal weight. For instance, if you're a wrestler who weighs 108 pounds and you need to get up to 113 pounds before the beginning of the season, create a timeline and plan to get there. Using our general rule of 0.5 to 1 pound per week with a goal of putting on an additional 5 pounds means it would take between 5 and 10 weeks to hit your weight gain goal. If your goal is gradual weight gain, begin by adding an additional 250 to 500 calories per day to your nutrition plan. If you're on target, great. If you're gaining weight too slowly, incrementally add 100 to 200 additional calories per day until you hit your target. If you're gaining weight too quickly, reduce your calories by 100 to 200 per day until you're on track.

Sometimes life throws us a curve ball, and we can't follow as gradual a plan as we would like. Whether it's from a lack of planning or simply your team needing you in a different spot, there will always be situations where you need to get results faster, even if the timing isn't ideal. In these cases, go as slowly as possible while still reaching for your goal. An additional 500 calories per day is estimated to add approximately 1 pound of weight per week, so see where you're sitting and adjust your plan accordingly.

Tip: What should you do if you can't seem to keep weight on? For some athletes, it can seem like an impossible task to keep weight on with all the activity they do throughout the week. In these cases, adding energy-dense foods throughout the day can help get in more calories without having to eat a much larger volume of food. Try adding foods such as nuts, nut butters, seeds, olive oil, or avocado to your meals for a quick calorie boost. It's important to remember that you're not replacing any foods on your plan with these items, but rather adding them on top of your current plan.

WEIGHT MAINTENANCE

Weight maintenance can be just as tricky as setting a goal to lose or gain weight. Some weight class sports, such as wrestling and rowing, require athletes to sit at a specific weight the entire season while closely monitoring their weight to make sure the player is not over or under for a competition. Likewise, some athletes may just be conscious about their weight and want to keep track of where they stand. Whatever your reason, keep a few things in mind. If your body is still growing, then weight gain is quite normal and healthy, even if it is at a faster rate. While not entirely accurate for all athletes, a good starting point for how much weight someone gains is as follows: For men, every inch of growth above five feet adds approximately six pounds of body weight. For women, every inch they grow above five feet adds approximately five pounds. If you're unsure of where you fall on the growth curve for your body, it would be best to consult your pediatrician or doctor. However, for athletes that aren't currently growing and want to maintain weight, there are a few things you can do to help facilitate that:

1. Maintain consistency in your eating habits year-round. One of the biggest pitfalls for athletes is having an extremely regimented diet during the season followed by a few months of eating without any kind of plan at all. Instead, try to maintain consistency year-round by having a loose plan to follow even when you aren't competing.

2. Adjust how much fuel you're taking in based on how active you are. Be sure to include fueling sources based on exercise timing when heading to a practice, training, or game. However, if it's a rest day or a very light workout, those extra snacks and meals likely aren't necessary.

3. Listen to your hunger cues. It's important for any individual (athlete or not) to be in tune with how his or her body feels. If you're physically hungry, the worst thing you can do is restrict food. Likewise, if you're feeling pleasantly full, forcing a meal can make you feel sick instead of energized.

4. Check the scale periodically. If you're feeling very full, then you need to evaluate two different things: If you're able to easily maintain weight, then it may be that you don't need to force yourself to get in extra calories. On the flip side, if you're feeling full but know your weight is trending down because of the scale readings, it's important to change up what you're eating. Sometimes athletes don't feel as hungry, because exercise may curb their appetite in some cases. In situations like this, it's important to make sure you're getting in the right calories, even if you're not feeling hungry. Smoothies or homemade protein shakes made with nut butter, fruits, and a dairy or plant-based milk can be good choices in these situations, as liquid calories are often easier to consume than whole foods and won't keep athletes full as long as a typical meal would.

CHAPTER NINE

BARRIERS TO PERFORMANCE AND NUTRITIONAL HEALTH

IF IT WAS EASY, everyone would be doing it, right? The truth is, between work and school schedules, training times, and competitions that could require hours of travel time, staying on track with a performance nutrition plan throughout the year will definitely have its challenges. Some factors are easy to control, like setting up your environment for success and having healthy snacks and fruits around. Others may not be so simple. In this day and age, it's quite common for many athletes to have barriers, such as medical conditions or food allergies, that may require a lot of planning around mealtime. Not only this, a male athlete of the same height, weight, and medical background, playing the same sport and position, may have completely different needs from a female athlete. The majority of scientific research regarding athletes and performance nutrition has historically been conducted on male athletes. This means that, while we can make some correlations for women, the data and results cannot be extrapolated for women and they will have unique circumstances that change their nutrition requirements and planning.

BODY

As discussed earlier, nutrition is a critical component in keeping the body energized and operating at 100 percent for every training session or tournament. However, a huge number of other factors come into play to keep the body performing well. Some factors are in your control, such as getting enough sleep, practicing mindfulness and meditation to keep yourself mentally strong, and limiting alcohol consumption. Unfortunately, a number of factors are outside of your control. Understanding which factors can be controlled and which can't will help you formulate a plan to be as healthy and competitive as possible in any scenario.

HEALTH CONDITIONS

Many different health conditions can afflict an individual or athlete. Whether it's an allergy or immune-related disease, these conditions can impact anything from an athlete's immune system to his or her strength and endurance on the field. Some conditions have symptoms that can be treated with a specific nutrition plan, while others may require a change in environment or medication.

Allergies

Allergies can have a big impact on an athlete's performance and physical health, and can range from minor to severe. Allergies related to food, such as lactose or dairy intolerance or celiac disease, have a direct effect on inflammation and/or the body's immune system. Even trace amounts of gluten in a dish—or even gluten residue on a cooking pan—can cause a severe reaction for those with celiac disease. When a food allergen is ingested, the body mistakes the ingredient for a foreign invader, and it sends out a chemical called histamine to combat it. This can range from something mild, such as slight inflammation or bloating, all the way to a serious or potentially life-threatening reaction called anaphylaxis. At best, these symptoms will have a poor result on athletic performance and can affect energy levels, focus, and recovery time. At worse, an EpiPen or hospital visit can be required for a life-threatening reaction. Whether your allergy is food-related or not, the best way to get a handle on it is to control your environment as much as possible. If you have a food allergy, pack meals and snacks from home to have the most control over the ingredients. When eating out, be sure to let your friends, family, and coaches know of your eating restrictions so that they can plan accordingly. In some cases, it may be best to call a restaurant ahead of time and notify them of a food restriction to ensure they can accommodate you.

Asthma

Asthma is a condition that can severely affect or even cripple an athlete's performance and ability to train during a flare-up. Asthma itself is a condition in which airways become narrow and a large layer of mucus is produced. This can cause anything from minor difficulties breathing or coughing to more serious flare-ups that make it difficult to function on a daily basis. Asthma in general should be closely monitored by a doctor, but the side effects can certainly make life for an athlete difficult. An asthma flare-up can be exercise induced or can be triggered during cold or dry seasons. Exercise is likely impossible during a flare-up, so the best way to combat this is to monitor your signs and symptoms and stay alert to what specifically triggers your asthma so that you can adjust your treatment options and plans as necessary with your doctor and coach.

Autoimmune Diseases

Autoimmune diseases are a classification of health condition in which an individual's immune system begins attacking healthy cells. A number of different autoimmune diseases exist, including lupus, rheumatoid arthritis, and inflammatory bowel disease (IBD). Some autoimmune disease symptoms can be managed well with diet and/or medication, while others cannot. The one thing autoimmune diseases have in common for an athlete is that they often cause symptoms such as inflammation, fatigue, and swelling. During a flare-up, it can be extraordinarily difficult to even get to a practice or game, let alone compete at your best. Understanding what causes your condition's flare-ups, whether it be food, stress, or a different environmental stressor, can be the first step in creating a plan to minimize symptoms.

EATING DISORDERS

Eating disorders are a cluster of different disorders that affect an individual's eating patterns or reaction to food. While no one thing can trigger an eating disorder, many different treatment options exist, depending on the type and severity of the condition. Research is not definitive, but researchers speculate that athletes, especially those in weight-focused or aesthetic sports, are particularly vulnerable.

Since eating disorders do not typically resolve on their own, it is important to get support. A treatment team for an eating disorder typically includes a physician, a therapist or psychologist, and a registered dietitian. This trifecta is used to cover the medical, emotional, and nutritional treatment of an individual. Furthermore, the level of care someone needs will depend on the severity of the disorder. Some individuals with milder symptoms are able to successfully get outpatient treatment, while others with more severe symptoms or health concerns may require an in-patient level of care to get better. The most common eating disorders that young athletes are susceptible to include the following:

Anorexia Nervosa

Anorexia is a condition in which an individual has an extreme desire to lose weight. Those afflicted with anorexia may purposely restrict eating or not have an appetite. Complications can include severe weight loss or failure to hit appropriate weight or growth goals in youth. While many individuals who have been diagnosed with anorexia nervosa have altered body compositions, this is not the case for everyone. An individual can have anorexia but still appear to have a normal or typical weight.

Binge Eating Disorder

Binge eating disorder is characterized by eating extremely large amounts of food while suffering from a feeling of lack of control. In other words, those with binge eating disorder struggle to be able to stop eating, and they feel out of control. While everyone overeats on occasion, those with BED deal with this on an extreme and regular basis.

Bulimia Nervosa

Bulimia is a condition in which an individual has a distorted view of his or her body image and strives for weight loss or changes in body composition. Those with bulimia nervosa will often cycle between periods of overeating followed by periods of purging (vomiting) or restricting food.

SUBSTANCE ABUSE

When most athletes think of substance abuse, they may picture individuals who are battling a lifelong drug or alcohol addiction that has a debilitating effect on their lives. The truth, however, is that substance abuse can range from these extreme cases to mild cases, such as having a few extra alcoholic drinks throughout the week. Substance abuse for athletes is quite common and can have negative effects on both their health and performance goals.

Alcohol

Alcohol can have a huge impact on an athlete's performance and recovery attempts, depending on the degree and frequency of consumption. In general, alcohol use should be limited due to its detrimental health and performance effects. In athletes, alcohol consumption causes a myriad of symptoms. Studies have shown that frequent alcohol consumption can inhibit muscle growth and recovery, due to inhibiting protein synthesis. Alcohol can also cause dehydration because it is a diuretic. From a nutritional standpoint, alcohol actually depletes nutrient stores and can cause deficiencies in many B vitamins over time. As a fuel source, alcohol cannot be used efficiently by the body for energy during activities. Instead, alcohol is converted directly into fatty acids and stored as body fat. While it may not be realistic to completely abstain from alcohol if you are over the age of 21, you can adhere to a few guidelines to minimize performance declines. Avoid alcohol consumption the day of a training or practice and abstain from alcohol the day before a big tournament or competition. The last thing you need is to wake up the day of a big game feeling sluggish, bloated, and fatigued. When drinking alcohol, practice moderation. Try not to have more than 1 or 2 drinks in a night and, if possible, follow each alcoholic beverage with a glass of water to ensure that you replace some of the fluids you may be losing throughout the day or night.

Drugs

Recreational drugs have as many different symptoms and side effects as there are types. Drugs that act as a depressant, such as cannabis and opiates, can reduce lung capacity and slow down oxygen flow to the body. Not only will this have a detrimental effect on an athlete's energy availability, but it also can lead to issues like difficulty concentrating and delayed reaction times. Unlike alcohol, drug use is illegal and therefore has no governing body ensuring that what you're using is even the substance you believe it to be. Drugs you believe are harmless could be laced with other unknown chemicals. Furthermore, athletes that undergo drug testing need to be particularly wary as there is an increased risk for testing positive on a banned substance list. The last thing a serious athlete wants to do is take him- or herself out of a game or get expelled from their sport because of a drug incident.

SLEEP DEPRIVATION

One thing that is often elusive to young athletes is proper rest. Trying to juggle class time, training, homework, social lives, and the occasional out-of-town competition can make it easy for sleep to fall to the wayside. Most young adults need eight to ten hours of sleep per night, while older athletes ideally want to get between seven and nine hours. Unfortunately, up to one-third of all athletes do not hit their sleep goals. Since sleep is required for many normal bodily functions, it's no wonder that inadequate sleep has some pretty dramatic side effects. Lack of sleep causes unfavorable shifts in the hormones that control the body's stress levels, alter hunger cues, and decrease satiety levels. In short, this means an individual is more likely to overeat throughout the day if he or she isn't getting adequate rest. Furthermore, sleep deprivation can impair the body's ability to repair skeletal muscle, thus having a potentially detrimental effect on both strength and recovery efforts. Finally, the most common symptom of sleep deprivation is fatigue. A sleep-deprived athlete will never be able to trump a well-rested player of the same caliber.

Luckily, you have a few simple ways to improve sleeping habits and the overall time and quality of your sleep, even with a busy schedule.

1. Set a consistent time to be in bed by. It can be hard for the body to adjust if you go to bed at 1:00 a.m. one night and 11:00 p.m. the next. The more consistent your schedule, the easier it will be to fall asleep.

2. Create a bedtime routine. Whether that's washing your face, reading a book, or journaling, a bedtime routine can help create consistency and build healthy sleep habits.

3. Limit screen time before bed. The blue light emitted from screens and phones has been shown to delay the production of melatonin, a chemical that helps induce sleep. Putting away phones and shutting off the TV an hour before bed can go a long way toward improving sleep quality.

4. If you must look at a screen, take precautions. Wear glasses that filter blue light as a decent substitution when screen time is inevitable.

5. Avoid caffeine after 12:00 p.m. Caffeine has a half-life of six hours. This means that six hours after ingestion, half of the caffeine is still circulating in our body. Avoiding caffeine doesn't just mean not drinking coffee or tea

after noon. It also means avoiding pre-workout sources of caffeine that are often found in energy drinks or formulas specifically marketed as workout enhancers.

MIND

In sports, the mental game can be just as important as physical performance when it comes to beating out the competition. And while nutrition is imperative to gaining a competitive edge, the difference between a win or loss can be determined by a battle of wills. When athletes have self-esteem issues or lack self-confidence in their game, it can pose challenges. Nerves can make a star player miss an easy shot or cause a veteran goalie to suddenly miss a point-blank catch. On the other end of mental battles are athletes who suffer from anxiety and diagnosed mental illnesses. Depression and other mental battles can make it extremely difficult for an athlete to perform his or her best. Some days athletes may feel at 100 percent, while other days they are barely able to get out of bed. Couple this with the pressure that athletes face about not letting the team or fellow athletes down. This can create a huge amount of stress on an athlete's physical and mental health. Mental illness among athletes isn't often talked about, but these issues affect athletes just as much as the average population.

BODY IMAGE

Body image issues are extremely common among athletes, especially those undergoing puberty. Changes in body composition that affect physical appearance can make even the toughest athlete sensitive. Women will often have increases in body fat, while men will begin to develop lean muscle mass. This change can leave women feeling particularly vulnerable during puberty. Meanwhile, men may feel uncomfortable prior to puberty if their peers have already begun seeing changes. Having a poor body image not only creates feelings of unrest, but also can potentially lead to patterns of disordered eating if one tries too hard to change his or her appearance (page 90). Moreover, having a poor body image can wreak havoc during a game. If thoughts about your body image or confidence levels begin to seep into everyday activities like training or being on the court, those negative feelings could subconsciously affect your play. Being confident in your own skin isn't something that comes naturally for many due to societal pressure and unrealistic standards of beauty and strength. But this doesn't mean that it has to be difficult. Focus each day on what you love about your body, whether it is being able to run several miles without getting winded, having the strength to be active for 14 or 16 hours a day without fail, or just acknowledging that as an individual, you have something unique to offer the world. If you focus on being comfortable in your skin, no matter your shape or size, you can go a long way toward not only being mentally confident, but also physically assertive on the field. If you're struggling with where to start, make a goal to look in the mirror every day for the next week and name one thing about yourself that you love.

FOCUS

Whether athletes are able to focus will dictate how and when they respond to both internal and external events during a game, competition, or even practice. Each sport may require varying levels of concentration based on both the player and setting. For example, a football player may need to focus on surveying the field to make the best call about a play for his team, and a wrestler may need to focus on opponents' weak points or look for breaks in their defense to discover the best way to overpower them. On a simpler scale, focus may also mean getting rid of distractions during a training session, such as putting a phone away or turning music off in order to hear the coach. Whatever form of focus an athlete may need in the moment, having the ability and training to concentrate on the moment at hand will go a long way in improving any athlete's mental and physical game.

Here are a few tips to help you train yourself to focus better:

1. Identify cues to look for based on your sport. Are you trying to find an opening to pass a ball to your teammate, surveying uneven terrain to avoid a sprain, or observing another team to look for openings in their defense? Identify which cues are important based on your sport.

2. Determine what obstacles make you lose focus. Are you distracted by technology or a material item? Do nerves make you lose focus when a play goes wrong? Does something trigger you when hearing your coach yelling by the sidelines? Identify the biggest obstacles that affect your focus.

3. Come up with a strategy. Once you've identified the roadblocks to your focus, come up with a strategy to overcome them. Whether it's meditation

or a mantra to pull yourself back to the moment, consciously identifying why certain things make you lose focus, or changing your environment for a better outcome, find methods to overcome these obstacles. The longer you work on implementing a strategy, the easier focusing will become.

CONSIDERATIONS FOR FEMALE ATHLETES

Competitive female athletes have unique energy and nutritional challenges. In addition to eating in order to maximize performance and recovery, women must consume the proper amount of calories and nutrition to maintain hormone levels, a proper menstrual cycle, and subsequent proper bone mineral density. A caloric intake that is too low or that does not take into account energy being burned from training needs can lead female athletes to have irregular periods or stop getting them altogether. While this might sound like a benefit to some, losing your period due to inadequate energy intake leads to fatigue and hormonal disruption, and it puts female athletes at an increased risk for stress fractures as well as osteopenia and osteoporosis in the future.

PREMENSTRUAL SYNDROME

Menstrual cycles can affect women, especially athletes, in many different ways. Prior to menstruation, many women will undergo Premenstrual Syndrome, or PMS for short. This typically starts five to eleven days before the beginning of a period and can have a range of effects on a female athlete, including cramping, headaches, fatigue, bloating, and water retention. Some female athletes will have more severe reactions and may be classified with Premenstrual Dysphoric Disorder (PMDD), amplifying both the symptoms and severity of PMS. For individuals with PMDD, severe anxiety, irritability, and depression are extremely common in addition to the physical symptoms. These symptoms affect female athletes in different ways, causing minor fatigue in some while being completely debilitating to others. Some female athletes undergoing PMS or PMDD will have a difficult time simply getting out of bed, let alone performing on the field. Symptoms typically go away once menstruation begins.

IRON DEFICIENCY

From a nutritional perspective, female athletes also lose a significant amount of iron during menstruation due to blood loss. This puts female athletes more at risk for low iron levels or iron deficiency anemia, which can cause extreme fatigue, weakness, and anxiousness. To combat this, female athletes should eat foods rich in iron, such as meat and poultry, spinach, tofu, lentils, eggs, and quinoa, to help keep iron stores at normal levels.

FEMALE ATHLETE TRIAD (RED-S)

In general, being an active woman who regularly gets exercise by participating in sports is a healthy behavior or habit. And while exercise typically has health benefits, such as improved mood and energy levels, some women may actually experience negative effects when their body's energy and nutritional needs are not being met. A common condition that exclusively affects female athletes is called the Female Athlete Triad (now known as Relative Energy Deficiency in Sport, or RED-S). The Female Athlete Triad is a cluster of conditions that occur when the body has low energy availability and isn't able to maintain normal physiological functioning. These symptoms include disordered eating, amenorrhea, and osteoporosis. Some women may experience all three symptoms, while others are only affected by one or two of these conditions.

DISORDERED EATING

Disordered eating is technically any eating pattern at a given time that is not normal. This includes things such as overeating, food or texture avoidance, or purposely restricting food for a short period of time. Every single human being experiences bouts of disordered eating at certain points in their lives. An athlete may forget to pack a snack during a long road trip to an away game and end up overeating later in the day because of her hunger. Certain young adults may have very specific food preferences and texture issues that cause them to only eat a specific set of foods on most days. In the case of the Female Athlete Triad, however, disordered eating is typically associated with not meeting minimum calorie and energy requirements throughout the day to maintain normal bodily function. Whether calories are being purposely restricted to lose weight or an athlete is simply underestimating their calorie needs based on their physical activity, this type of disordered eating can lead to low energy availability in the body. And since menstrual cycles require a certain level of energy needs in order to function properly, low energy availability can lead to irregular or completely stopped periods.

AMENORRHEA

Often caused by low energy availability or hormonal disruptions in the body, amenorrhea is characterized by the loss of a woman's monthly menstrual cycle. While not having to deal with a monthly menstrual cycle may sound appealing to some, this loss actually wreaks havoc on the body and can affect not only short-term, but also long-term health. Because part of the menstrual cycle involves producing estrogen and progesterone, two hormones related to building strong bones, when the period disappears, bones begin to become weak or brittle.

OSTEOPOROSIS

Following amenorrhea is the risk of developing soft or weak bones that are prone to fractures. It's not a coincidence that stress fractures are particularly common among female athletes. When amenorrhea causes hormonal disruptions, young female athletes are at risk for an early onset of health conditions related to their bone density. Building strong bones is similar to storing money in a bank account at a young age. Between the ages of 9 and 19, the majority of an individual's bone density is formed. Once someone hits the age of 30, they slowly begin to lose their bone density. Osteoporosis, which is a condition where an individual has extremely weak or porous bones, can affect athletes as early as their teenage years, and it is not reversible. This means these athletes will be prone to stress fractures and other bone-related diseases for the rest of their lives. Osteoporosis affects not just their ability to perform in sports, but their long-term health as well.

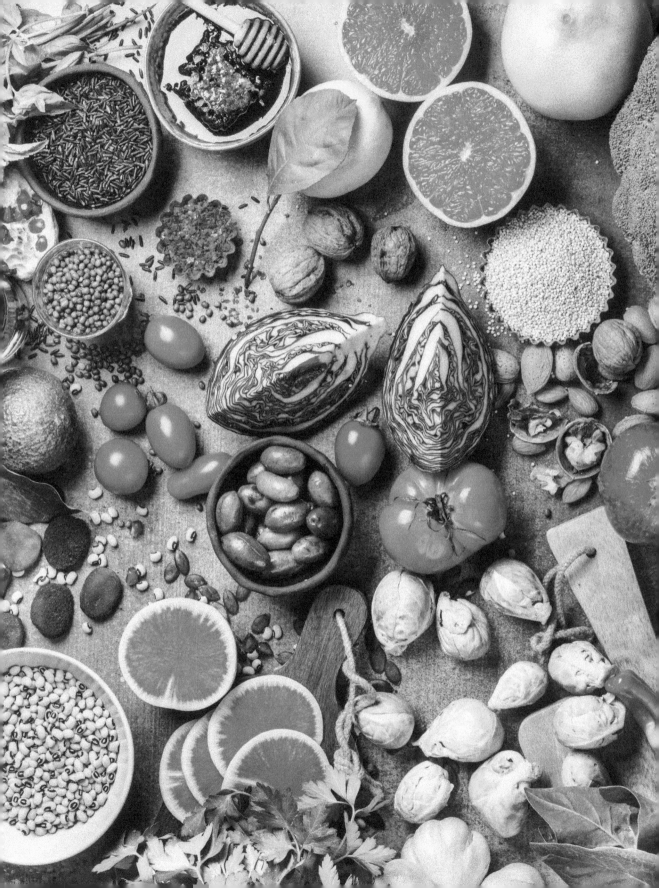

CHAPTER TEN

USING NUTRITION TO FUEL RECOVERY

PROPER NUTRITION NOT ONLY HELPS athletes recover on a daily basis from the demands of training, but it also plays a huge role in recovering from injury. The right performance plan can reduce inflammation and even speed up recovery in some cases by providing the proper nutrients and energy needed to help the body optimize healing. Conversely, a poor nutrition plan can lead to losses of lean muscle mass, weight gain, and can even extend the amount of time it takes for you to get back into the gym or onto the field.

REHABILITATION

When the body is rehabilitating from injury, it is under a large amount of stress. Not only is inflammation present, but the body is rebuilding and remodeling damaged tissues and/or bones. On top of this, an athlete may be undergoing physical therapy or rehab in order to facilitate treatment. By providing the right balance of energy, fluids, protein, and micronutrients, an athlete can supply the building blocks the body needs to optimize its repair and recovery time. The goal of a recovery nutrition plan for athletes is to support tissue growth and repair, preserve muscle mass, and balance energy needs during a change in physical activity.

INFLAMMATION

Inflammation is a defense mechanism by the human body in response to an injury, and it can last for several days after an incident. During inflammation, the body releases several chemicals to combat any foreign or dangerous substances. While inflammation is a normal process, it's not something you want for a prolonged period of time. Inflammation causes redness, swelling, pain, and decreased movement or flexibility in the area of the injury. Luckily, you have plenty of anti-inflammatory foods to choose from in order to help fight inflammation and speed up the healing process. Foods rich in vitamins A, C, and D have anti-inflammatory properties. Try choosing foods such as tomatoes, citrus, cantaloupe, red and green peppers, carrots, and dark leafy greens to give a boost of anti-inflammatory properties to the body. Additionally, the omega-3 fatty acids found in fatty fish such as salmon or tuna are known for their anti-inflammatory properties and can help speed up healing.

MUSCLE SORENESS

Most injuries involve a degree of tissue damage that the body needs to spend time repairing. This process can take just days, or can be more serious and require weeks or even months to fully heal. In order for the body to do its job, it needs the proper materials in its arsenal. Foods rich in high-quality protein will aid tissue repair and recovery. Make sure your diet is full of high-quality protein sources such as lean poultry (chicken or turkey), low-fat Greek yogurt or cottage cheese, nuts, and legumes to help the body meet its increased protein needs during tissue rebuilding.

Tip: There is a fine line between providing the body with enough calories and nutrition to support the healing process and overconsuming calories, which may put on a significant amount of body fat during an injury. While an injured body does have slightly increased needs compared to baseline energy requirements, an athlete on injury rest is often significantly less active during this time, possibly even completely sedentary. This means the athlete likely needs to dial back on total calorie consumption. Even participating in physical therapy or therapeutic exercise is likely much less strenuous energy-wise compared to a regular practice or training session. Being aware of your food intake and choosing foods that support healing versus those that are so-called empty and potentially pro-inflammatory (e.g., red meats, fried food, bakery items) is a good first step in fueling the body optimally for recovery.

INJURY

Injuries can come in many forms and for many different reasons: An athlete may not warm up properly and receive a sprain during activity; may be training too frequently and acquire an injury from overuse; or potentially may have a more serious occurrence in which a bone is fractured or broken due to play time or there is an accident on the field. Whatever the reason, injuries should be closely monitored by a professional and a treatment plan should be put in place immediately to avoid aggravation of the injury and speed up recovery time. Here are some of the most common sports injuries:

ACL sprain or tear: A tear or sprain in a ligament that helps stabilize the knee.

Concussion: A hit or blow to the head, causing the brain to be bruised or shaken.

Groin pull: More common in men, a strain to the groin muscles, often due to a lack of flexibility.

Shin splints: Often found in endurance runners, shin splints are characterized by pain in the lower leg bone and can occur when increasing running distance or frequency too quickly.

Tennis or golf elbow: Inflammation in the tendons surrounding the forearm, often caused by overuse or a repetitive movement that puts strain on the area.

Whatever the injury type or cause, all injuries are extremely serious, and you should seek immediate medical attention. Let your coach and athletic trainer know immediately when an injury has occurred so that it can be checked out as soon as possible. What might seem like a minor injury could turn into something more serious if left untreated and may even require surgery in some cases.

IMMUNE HEALTH

Immune health in young athletes is a complicated topic. Some studies have shown that regular exercise and activity helps strengthen the body's immune response and protect against sickness, while others have shown that intense activity, particularly endurance sports, may put the body at an increased risk. Regardless of the literature, it is extremely important for young athletes to have a strong immune system if they want to be competitive in their sport. A strong immune system can be the difference between rarely getting sick and having to miss practices and matches several times per year due to being bedridden. So how do athletes keep their immune systems up? Besides having proper hygiene and hand-washing behaviors, nutrition plays a significant role in the body's ability to fight off infections.

VIRAL INFECTIONS

Viral infections, such as a cold or upper respiratory infection, happen when the body's immune system is not strong enough to fight off the infection. Factors such as physical or mental stress from long practice hours, school work, and inadequate sleep can contribute to a weakened immune system. Proper nutrition and hydration improve the body's ability to fight off infections as well as aid in the recovery process when an athlete is already sick. Eating foods that are high in protein and contain vitamins A, C, E, D, and zinc has been shown to protect an athlete's immune system and help fight back against infection. Proper hydration is also extremely important for a functioning immune system. Water helps remove toxins from the body, and inadequate fluid intake could make the body more susceptible to an attack.

Creating a game plan that includes the right nutrition and hydration, stress reduction, and adequate sleep can go a long way in fighting off illness. The next time you're under a large amount of stress or fighting off an infection, try the following:

Consume immune-boosting foods. Anti-inflammatory and immune-boosting foods, such as fruits, vegetables, legumes, nuts, low-fat dairy, and foods high in vitamin D, such as fortified milk or plant-based milks, fortified grains, egg yolks, and fatty fish, can help the body fight off infection.

Stay hydrated. Drink adequate fluids when sick to remove toxins from the body and reduce symptoms of an illness. Even if practice is not in the cards, aim to get in a minimum of eight to ten cups of water throughout the day to keep the body properly hydrated.

Practice stress reduction. Whether it's coming up with a plan for when to fit in school work and studying, meditating, practicing yoga, or just setting time to relax during the day, reducing stress has a significant impact on keeping the immune system healthy.

Have a sleep schedule. Poor sleep habits can lead to a suppressed immune system and put the body more at risk for getting an illness. Aim to get seven to nine hours of sleep every night at a minimum, and try to get ready for bed at roughly the same time every night when possible.

GUT MICROBIOME

Having a healthy gut means having a healthy and strong immune system. When most people think of the gut, they simply think of the digestive process their food undergoes. But recent research has discovered that the gut is actually responsible for much more in the human body. Within your gut is something called a microbiome, which can consist of billions of different bacteria that are either friendly or harmful. When the gut microbiome is strong, the friendly bacteria act like little soldiers, creating a solid defense in the body and strengthening the immune system against foreign invaders. When your gut health is poor or there is an influx of harmful bacteria, the body's defenses are weakened and it's left open to attack. Recent research has further linked gut health to many conditions, including depression, food intolerances, acne, and you guessed it, immune health. Focusing on foods that help support the gut microbiome and stomach lining can help protect the body from illness. Foods high in soluble fiber can provide fuel to the good bacteria in your gut and supercharge your defenses. These include foods such as fruits, vegetables, whole-grain oatmeal or rice, lentils, chickpeas, and seeds. Fermented foods such as pickles, have also been shown to be an excellent fuel source for the gut. Next time you're feeling adventurous, add some sauerkraut, kimchi, or kefir to your meal or snack.

Antibiotics and Athletes

Antibiotics are a type of drug used to help the body ward off diseases and infections caused specifically by bacteria. If an athlete has a bacteria-based infection, these drugs can help quash an infection and get an athlete back to health in a matter of days. Unfortunately, there is a big caveat when it comes to taking antibiotics. The more often an individual uses antibiotics to ward off a bacterial infection, the more the body builds a resistance to these drugs. For this reason, it's always best to consult your doctor when you feel ill to see if and when antibiotics are warranted.

In addition to wiping out bacteria that cause infections, antibiotics can also wipe out the good bacteria that live in the gut and contribute to digestive health. To combat this, taking a quality probiotic with a variety of different strains can help replenish the good bacteria in the gut. When looking at probiotics, choose products that require refrigeration and that have several million different active live cultures.

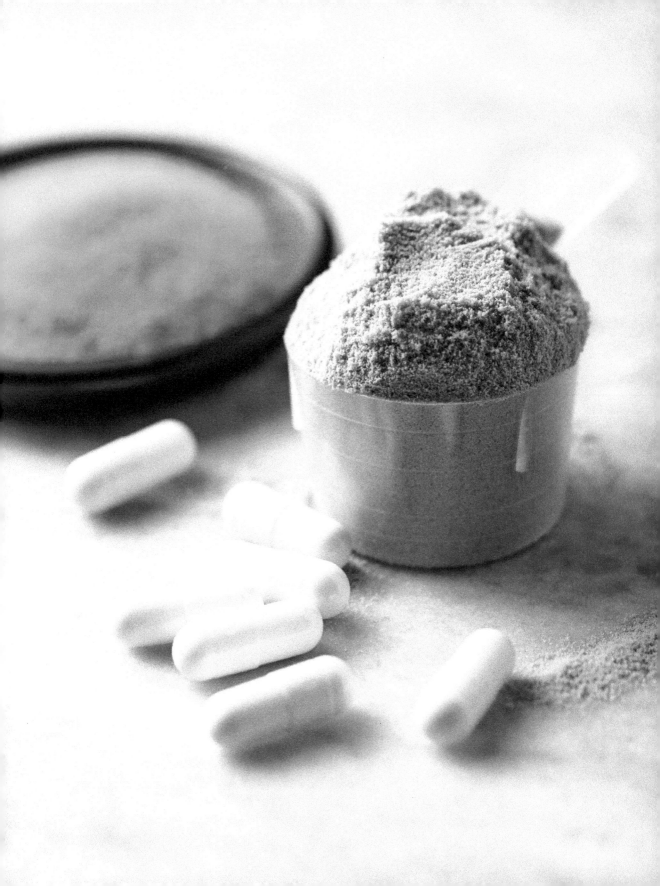

CHAPTER ELEVEN

PERFORMANCE ENHANCERS AND SUPPLEMENTS

AS A SPORTS DIETITIAN, the question I get asked the most by young adults and athletes alike has to do with supplements. With the media touting supplements as the solution to everything from increasing energy to enhancing strength, shortening recovery, and helping the body burn fat, it's no wonder that so many athletes are confused. Supplements come in all shapes and sizes—literally, they are anything that "supplements" the diet. They can be vitamins and minerals, sports drinks, protein powders, or performance-enhancing products. While some supplements can be beneficial or at the very worst harmless, others can have negative performance and health effects or can be downright dangerous, such as with anabolic steroids. To make matters more complicated, some supplements are banned from sports by the NCAA, and if an athlete unknowingly consumes a product with one of these ingredients, it could jeopardize his or her spot on the team. This chapter will discuss the potential benefits and risks of common supplements in the athletic world, but it's important that any athlete considering a supplement consult his or her doctor, coach, and athletic trainer prior to adding one to their regimen.

DIETARY SUPPLEMENTS

Most athletes have varying opinions of what is considered a dietary supplement. Some may picture vitamins, while others consider sports drinks or even performance-enhancing powders to be supplements. In reality, any type of nutrition obtained outside of foods and natural beverages is considered a dietary supplement. This section will discuss the most common types of supplements and what to consider before adding one to a regimen.

IRON

Iron is a mineral that helps athletes have proper energy stores and a strong immune system. It is typically found in foods such as nuts, spinach, meat, and fortified cereals and grains. Female athletes tend to be more at risk for an iron deficiency due to iron losses each month during menstrual periods. If considering a supplement, iron should always be taken with food as iron by itself can be harsh on the stomach and cause stomach distress.

CALCIUM

This mineral is needed for proper bone health and muscle contractions in active young adults and athletes alike. Food sources of calcium include fortified animal milk, fortified plant milk, cheese, yogurt, dark leafy greens, dried fruit, and tofu. If an athlete's diet does not contain dairy, a supplement may be necessary. Aim for roughly 1,000 to 1,300 milligrams of calcium a day. When choosing supplements, always try to get one that contains both calcium and vitamin D, as both are needed together for proper absorption into the body.

VITAMIN D

Also called the sunshine vitamin, vitamin D is responsible for a number of functions in the body, including bone health, a strong immune system, mood stability, and energy regulation. Like calcium, vitamin D is predominantly found in fortified milk or plant milks, as well as in fatty fish, oranges, and eggs. If an athlete doesn't regularly get these foods and they're not exposed to at least fifteen minutes of sunshine per day, a supplement may be necessary. Aim for supplements that have 400 to 600 IU of vitamin D3 in them to help meet daily needs. If you have a vitamin D deficiency, consult your doctor or dietitian for therapeutic amounts.

VITAMIN B12

Vitamin B12 is necessary for energy production throughout the body. Athletes who have extremely low stores can develop vitamin B12 anemia. Since B12 is predominantly found in animal products, such as meat, poultry, fish, eggs, milk, and yogurt, vegetarians and vegans are typically at high risk for deficiencies. Adults need approximately 2.4 micrograms of B12 daily. Be wary of supplements with ingredient blends, however, as many powders, energy drinks, and pre-workout supplements will often have double or even quadruple the needed amount of B12.

SPORTS DRINKS

As discussed in the hydration section (page 16), sports drinks are extremely popular with athletes. While some marketing would have the average, non-athletic person believing that sports drinks are beneficial for everyone, typically only athletes that need to replace fluids, electrolytes, and glycogen at the same time will benefit. Athletes who work out in hot or humid conditions, are heavy sweaters, or who engage in moderate activity for an hour or longer on a regular basis will likely benefit from a sports drink that contains carbohydrates, sodium, potassium, and fluids. Sports drinks can help an endurance runner or cyclist have consistent energy levels throughout a race, or can provide a quick fuel source during a competition when an athlete otherwise wouldn't have a chance to sit down and eat a food-based snack. Unlike most supplements, as long as sports drinks don't contain any additional vitamins, minerals, or performance-enhancing ingredients, they tend to be a relatively safe fuel source for most physically active athletes who undergo prolonged periods of exercise.

PROTEIN DRINKS

Protein powders and shakes are one of the most commonly used supplements among athletes, and for good reason: They're a convenient and easy way to meet protein needs throughout the day, especially right after a practice or workout.

There are, however, many factors that influence whether an athlete should consume a protein shake and, if so, what type of powder or shake they should use. In most situations, athletes will get enough protein from food sources such as dairy, meats, poultry, and fish, while meeting their daily needs. Additionally, whole-food sources of protein don't just contain protein. They often include other beneficial nutrients that help fuel the body and repair muscles after a long practice. For this reason, it is recommended to get in food sources of protein whenever possible. However, this isn't always possible or easy, and in certain situations a protein supplement can be beneficial—for example, right after a practice or workout when there is a long car ride home or a lack of food options available. In these situations, make sure that your protein powder either has 45 to 60 grams of quick-digesting carbohydrates, or pair a low-carbohydrate protein powder with a carbohydrate source such as milk or fruit. Additionally, there are different forms of protein powder and not all are created equal. Here are the most common protein powder types:

Whey Protein Isolate

This is a high-quality, rapidly digesting protein. Whey protein isolate is recommended when consuming a protein shake or powder after a workout or training, as it is rapidly absorbed by the body and can begin repairing muscle tissue immediately.

Whey Protein Concentrate

Whey protein concentrate is a lower-quality whey protein that is not absorbed as well as whey protein isolate. It can often be found in premade shakes or bars. When possible, choose whey protein isolate over concentrate.

Casein Powder

Casein is a slow-digesting protein powder that takes longer for the body to absorb. For this reason, it isn't recommended as a post-workout protein source.

POLYPHENOL SUPPLEMENTS

Polyphenols have many health benefits, but a major one is their powerful antioxidant properties. Since polyphenols are found predominantly in plant-based foods, having a diet that includes apples, berries, grapes, spinach, broccoli, carrots, and dark chocolate is an excellent way to get a power punch of polyphenols into the body and help fight inflammation. Polyphenols from food sources are safe to consume in virtually any amount because of the specific content of this chemical that is found in foods. Unfortunately, that isn't the case with supplements. Many products on the market tout polyphenols as the next big supplement, and they may have hundreds of thousands of times the amount of polyphenols than are naturally found in foods. The best way to explain how poly-phenols work is to relate them to a pinball machine. In pinball, you want to hit certain targets in order to score points. Polyphenols work in a similar way: You want them to target specific components in the body called free radicals in order to neutralize them and the inflammation that comes with them. But what would happen if your pinball machine was suddenly spitting out dozens or hundreds of balls? All of your targets would get hit, but the massive influx of balls in the machine would begin wreaking havoc in other ways, likely breaking the machine and causing damage in the process. The same is true with polyphenols. Too many polyphenols at one time can turn them from being anti-inflammatory to pro-inflammatory. For this reason, it's best to get polyphenol sources from whole foods and leave the supplements on the shelf.

SPECIALIZED PERFORMANCE SUPPLEMENTS

Performance enhancing supplements make some pretty catchy claims. Getting bigger, stronger, faster, and more energized simply by taking a pill or powder is enough to tempt any athlete to try one of the thousands of supplements on the market. And while supplements have a place in an athlete's tool kit, the majority of products on the market are ineffective at best and dangerous at worst. Ath-letes who undergo drug testing need to be especially careful when choosing to take a supplement, as a seemingly harmless product could be contaminated with trace amounts of a substance banned by the NCAA. Nevertheless, a handful of well-researched supplements have been proven to benefit performance in certain athletes. Since supplement studies typically only look at adult partici-pants, there is little to no data on how different supplements affect young-adult athletes. It is impossible to know if an ingredient or product can have adverse reactions on growth or other health-related markers of a younger population. Therefore, the discussion about supplement types in this section only applies to individuals who are eighteen years or older.

AMINO ACIDS

Amino acids—particularly the branched-chain amino acids (BCAAs) found in meat, eggs, fish, poultry, and dairy—play an important role in building protein and muscle tissue. They are used as an energy source during activity, and even reduce exercise-related muscle tissue damage. Unfortunately, the data regarding BCAA supplements is unclear. While some studies do show that these benefits translate during supplement use, others have found that too many BCAAs from supplements can actually delay recovery time by blocking other proteins from being absorbed by the body. Choosing food sources over a supplement form of BCAAs may be a safer bet in getting both the performance- and recovery-related benefits and ensuring that an athlete is helping, not harming, his or her competitive edge.

CAFFEINE

Caffeine is a stimulant found in supplement form and in many foods and beverages, including coffee, tea, and energy drinks. Caffeine has been studied in the adult athletic population for its benefits related to fatigue reduction as well as the rate of perceived exertion during endurance events. Athletes report that caffeine effects vary greatly from one person to the next. While some individuals may feel alert and awake with a small amount of caffeine, others may feel jittery or anxious. The general dosage for adult athletes taking caffeine during an endurance event is 3 to 6 milligrams per kilogram of body weight. Note that consuming caffeine after 12:00 p.m. has been linked to difficulty sleeping. Also, caffeine in amounts greater than 15 micrograms per milliliter (roughly 500 milligrams) is considered a banned substance according to the NCAA, so athletes should be very careful when deciding if and when to use caffeine as a performance aid.

CREATINE

Creatine can either be taken in from food sources or as a supplement in the form of creatine monohydrate. This supplement has been linked to improved muscular strength and athletic performance during intense training sessions, particularly by those who engage in resistance training or weight-bearing exercises. Due to the immense research surrounding creatine, it is one of the few supplements on the market that is deemed generally safe for adult consumption.

If you're an adult athlete looking to use creatine, one of the best times to use this supplement is in the off-season while working on building strength. The general recommended dosage for creatine is to take 20 grams of creatine monohydrate for five days, followed by 5 grams for five to eight weeks.

L-CARNITINE

L-carnitine is an amino acid naturally produced by the body. Because L-carnitine levels drop during intense exercise, some supplement manufacturers have speculated about its use as a fat burner or energy-enhancing aid. L-carnitine is frequently added to energy drinks or pre-workout formulas for this reason. Unfortunately, the majority of research analyzing L-carnitine has shown insignificant results as a performance enhancer in adult athletes.

BLOWING THE WHISTLE ON STEROIDS AND OTHER PEDS

Steroids and other performance enhancing drugs (PEDs), such as human growth hormone (HGH) and prohormones, are artificially produced hormones and chemicals that are used to increase muscle mass and testosterone levels in adult athletes. In sports, the purpose is to improve athletic performance. However, steroids and PEDs are considered foul play in the world of athletics and have been banned due to their unfair performance advantage. The use of these banned substances is called "doping," and dedicated anti-doping organizations, including the United States Anti-Doping Agency (USADA), have been established to enforce these regulations. Besides risking expulsion from a sport, use of steroids and PEDs have been linked to a variety of side effects, including acne, excessive and abnormal body hair growth, intense mood swings, increased risk for heart attacks, and even stunted growth in youth athletes. Sexual development can also be affected, including breast development in men and facial hair growth in women. The potential risks of taking PEDs far outweigh any benefit an athlete would gain from taking these substances.

PART IV

Game-Winning Recipes

NOW THAT YOU HAVE A BETTER understanding of the factors that impact your nutritional and performance needs, let's get into some specific recipes that may help you on your journey to maximizing your performance potential. The recipes in this book are designed to give you a balanced plate of carbohydrates, protein, and fats, depending on your competition needs, all without sacrificing flavor. The chapters are broken down according to pregame, game day, and postgame recovery in order to provide you with some easy options during each phase of competition. You will also find a section dedicated to making quick and simple sports drinks. Pick some of your favorite-sounding recipes, spend an hour or two in the kitchen, and gear yourself for success while getting some delicious meals in as well.

CHAPTER TWELVE

PREGAME RECIPES

FOCUSING ON PERFORMANCE NUTRITION is important all season long, but especially so the day before a competition. Foods that are rich in carbohydrates with a balance of proteins and fats will help keep muscle glycogen stores topped off while ensuring that your body gets the proper nutrition it needs to stay strong. Pregame day meals should be consumed like any other day, with a focus on balanced meals spread evenly throughout the day based on your school, work, and training schedule. If you are going to practice, be sure to include pre- and post-workout fueling as well to remain consistent.

Southwest Skillet Omelet

YIELD: Serves 1 **PREP TIME:** 10 minutes **COOK TIME:** 10 minutes

This delicious omelet provides a mix of quality protein, starchy carbohydrates, and a powerful punch of vegetables that will help keep you fueled all morning long.

1 tablespoon olive oil
½ cup diced sweet potato
¼ cup pinto or black beans
¼ cup chopped red peppers

2 scallions, green parts only,
  thinly sliced
2 large eggs
2 egg whites

Salt and pepper to taste
⅛ cup reduced-fat cheddar
  cheese, shredded

1. In a small sauté pan over medium-high heat, heat the oil until shimmering. Add the sweet potato, beans, and peppers and cook for 2 minutes. Add the scallions and cook for an additional minute.

2. While the vegetables are cooking, combine the eggs, egg whites, salt, and pepper in a medium bowl and whisk until well combined. Add the egg mixture to the pan and cook.

3. Once the edges of the omelet begin to set, lift them with a rubber spatula and tilt the pan to allow any liquid to go underneath. Cook the omelet for an additional 2 minutes or until the omelet has mostly set.

4. Carefully flip the omelet with a spatula. Sprinkle cheese over the omelet and fold in half. Cook for an additional 2 minutes. Serve.

Recipe Tips: To make this dish dairy-free, omit the cheese. If you don't have scallions on hand, swap them out with ⅓ cup chopped onions instead. Serve the omelet by itself or with whole-wheat toast or fruit, depending on carbohydrate and dietary needs.

Storage: This omelet is best eaten fresh, but it can be stored in the fridge for up to three days.

Nutritional Information: Calories: 483, Total Fat: 27g, Saturated Fat: 7g, Protein: 29g, Carbohydrates: 32g, Fiber: 6g, Sodium: 381mg

Cottage Cheese Pancakes

YIELD: Serves 4 **PREP TIME:** 5 minutes **COOK TIME:** 10 minutes

Cottage cheese and whole-wheat flour come together to give a makeover to traditional pancakes. This version is packed with protein and gets its sweetness naturally from a combination of fruit and honey.

1 cup low-fat cottage cheese

3 large eggs

2 tablespoons canola oil or butter, plus 2 teaspoons for coating

1 teaspoon vanilla extract

⅓ cup whole-wheat flour

½ tablespoon cinnamon

2 medium bananas, thinly sliced

1 tablespoon honey (optional)

1. In a medium mixing bowl, combine the cottage cheese, eggs, 2 tablespoons of oil or butter, and vanilla extract. Add the flour and cinnamon and stir until combined.

2. In a medium skillet over medium-low heat, heat 1 teaspoon of oil or butter. Using a ¼-cup measuring cup, pour batter into the skillet, leaving an inch of room between each pancake.

3. Cook for 2 minutes, or until bubbles appear on the surface of the pancakes. Flip carefully with a spatula and cook for an additional minute. Remove the cooked pancakes to a plate.

4. Repeat steps 2 and 3 with the remaining batter.

5. Top each serving of pancakes with banana slices and a drizzle of honey, if desired.

Recipe Tips: To make this recipe gluten-free or Paleo, replace the whole-wheat flour with ¼ cup almond flour (not almond meal) and 2 tablespoons coconut flour. If your batter is too dry, add an additional egg.

Storage: These pancakes keep fresh in the fridge for three days or can be stored in the freezer without the banana for up to three months. To freeze, place each individual pancake between a sheet of parchment paper and store in a freezer bag or container.

Nutritional Information: Calories: 272, Total Fat: 14g, Saturated Fat: 3g, Protein: 14g, Carbohydrates: 24g, Fiber: 3g, Sodium: 274mg

Very Berry Parfait

YIELD: Serves 1 **PREP TIME:** 5 minutes **COOK TIME:** 10 minutes

This parfait has such a delectable flavor and texture that you may feel like you're eating dessert for breakfast. The berries make this recipe rich in anti-oxidants and phytochemicals—the perfect meal for an athlete or endurance runner looking to recover from a long training or practice.

½ cup blueberries
½ cup strawberries, sliced
2 tablespoons honey
1 tablespoon water

¾ cup low-fat vanilla Greek yogurt (free of artificial sweeteners)
½ cup granola

1. In a medium saucepan over medium-low heat, combine the blueberries, strawberries, honey, and water. Cover and cook for 5 minutes, or until the berries begin to gel, stirring occasionally. Remove from heat.

2. In a small glass cup or bowl, layer half of the berry mixture, ½ cup of Greek yogurt, and ¼ cup granola. Repeat layers until the parfait is built.

Recipe Tips: To make this recipe dairy-free and vegetarian, use an almond-, soy-, or coconut-based yogurt. To make this vegan, also replace the honey with agave or maple syrup. To make this gluten-free and Paleo, omit the granola. Looking to add a boost of protein? Mix a half-scoop of whey protein isolate into the Greek yogurt before layering the parfait.

Storage: If not consuming right away, store the berry mixture and yogurt in separate containers in the fridge for up to 48 hours. Assemble right before serving.

Nutritional Information: Calories: 548, Total Fat: 6g, Saturated Fat: 2g, Protein: 21g, Carbohydrates: 113g, Fiber: 8g, Sodium: 102mg

White Chicken Chili

YIELD: Serves 6 (1-cup servings) **PREP TIME:** 20 minutes **COOK TIME:** 30 minutes

This chili recipe is packed with flavor despite being lighter than a traditional tomato-based recipe. The high fiber and protein will keep an athlete full while helping to repair muscle tissue.

1 rotisserie chicken (approximately 2 pounds)

1 tablespoon olive oil

1 (4-ounce) can chopped green chiles

1 jalapeño pepper, chopped

3 cloves garlic

2 teaspoons ground cumin

½ teaspoon chili powder

4 cups low-sodium chicken broth

6 scallions, chopped

⅓ cup chopped cilantro leaves, packed

2 (15-ounce) cans white beans

Salt and pepper to taste

3 cups cooked brown rice

1. On a cutting board, remove the skin from the chicken and cut or pull the meat off the bone. Cut the poultry into 1-inch cubes. Set aside.

2. In a large saucepan over medium heat, heat the oil until shimmering. Add the green chiles, jalapeño, garlic, cumin, and chili powder and cook for 2 minutes, stirring occasionally.

3. Stir in the chicken broth, scallions, and cilantro until all ingredients are well combined. Once the broth is heated through, add in the chicken and the beans. Increase heat to medium-high and cook until the liquid comes to a boil, stirring occasionally.

4. Reduce the heat to low and cover the pan. Allow the chili to simmer for 15 minutes, or until slightly thickened. Add salt and pepper to taste.

5. To serve, pour 1 cup of chili over half a cup of brown rice.

Recipe Tips: To make this dish vegetarian, use a vegetable broth, omit the chicken, and add in an additional 16-ounce can of white beans. For those with a gluten intolerance or allergy, be sure to check that the chicken broth used has a GF label.

Storage: The chili can be stored in the fridge for up to three days or placed in a freezer-safe container for up to three months.

Nutritional Information: Calories: 446, Total Fat: 15g, Saturated Fat: 4g, Protein: 32g, Carbohydrates: 50g, Fiber: 10g, Sodium: 1,191mg

Asian-Style Chicken Salad

YIELD: Serves 2 **PREP TIME:** 20 minutes

After you taste how delicious and refreshing this salad is, you'll wonder why you would ever order takeout. This recipe is full of nutrient-rich fruits and vegetables that will keep you energized all day long.

FOR THE DRESSING

2 cloves garlic, finely minced

½ cup low-sodium soy sauce or coconut aminos

1 tablespoon minced ginger

2 tablespoons honey

FOR THE SALAD

8 ounces cooked chicken breast or skinless rotisserie chicken, cut into 1-inch cubes

4 cups shredded romaine lettuce

2 cups shredded red or green cabbage

½ cup shredded carrots

¼ cup sliced almonds

3 scallions, chopped

2 clementines, peeled and split into sections

½ cup crunchy chow mein noodles (optional)

TO MAKE THE DRESSING

Mix together the garlic, soy sauce, ginger, and honey in a small bowl. Set aside.

TO MAKE THE SALAD

1. In a salad bowl or large mixing bowl, toss together the chicken, lettuce, cabbage, carrots, almonds, scallions, and clementines. Add in the dressing and continue to toss until the ingredients are gently coated.

2. If using the noodles, add to the salad right before serving.

Storage: This recipe will keep in the fridge for up to 48 hours. Simply place the dressing and clementine sections in separate containers from the rest of the ingredients and mix together before serving.

Nutritional Information: Calories: 403, Total Fat: 9g, Saturated Fat: 1g, Protein: 37g, Carbohydrates: 45g, Fiber: 8g, Sodium: 2,408mg

Veggie Quesadilla

YIELD: Serves 2 **PREP TIME:** 15 minutes **COOK TIME:** 10 minutes

These quesadillas are packed with so much flavor that they're a meal by themselves. Hearty black beans, cheese, and Greek yogurt come together to make this dish rich in protein. These quesadillas are perfect for a pregame lunch or postgame dinner.

1 tablespoon avocado or canola oil

½ cup chopped red bell pepper

½ small white onion, chopped

½ cup black beans, rinsed

1 clove garlic, minced

Salt and pepper to taste

1 (6-ounce) container plain Greek yogurt

½ lime, juiced

2 (12-inch) whole-wheat tortillas

½ cup shredded low-fat cheese

1 avocado, sliced (optional)

1. In a medium skillet over medium-high heat, heat the oil until shimmering. Add the bell pepper, onions, beans, garlic, salt, and pepper and cook for 3 to 4 minutes or until the vegetables begin to turn translucent, stirring occasionally.

2. While the vegetables are cooking, stir together the Greek yogurt and lime juice in a small bowl. Set aside.

3. Move the cooked vegetables to a medium bowl and clean the pan.

4. Return the clean pan back to the heat and place 1 tortilla in the pan. Top half of the tortilla with one-quarter cup cheese and half of the vegetable mixture. Fold the tortilla in half and let cook for 2 minutes, or until the bottom of the tortilla appears golden brown. Carefully flip the tortilla and cook the other side for an additional minute. Repeat with the remaining tortilla and ingredients.

5. Serve immediately with the yogurt mixture and avocado, if using.

Recipe Tip: To make this gluten-free, purchase gluten-free tortillas or use corn tortillas that are free of wheat.

Storage: The quesadillas are best eaten immediately but can be stored in the fridge for up to 24 hours. To reheat, place in a pan on low heat and cook for 5 minutes or until warmed through.

Nutritional Information: Calories: 475, Total Fat: 19g, Saturated Fat: 3g, Protein: 27g, Carbohydrates: 46g, Fiber: 7g, Sodium: 697mg

Skillet Meat Sauce with Spaghetti

YIELD: Serves 8 **PREP TIME:** 5 to 10 minutes **COOK TIME:** 40 minutes

Meat sauce has been a staple in my house since I was a kid and is one of my favorite dishes. Traditional meat sauce often takes hours to cook and is packed with oil and fat. Luckily, this dish is much quicker to cook and is full of veggies instead of fat, but still has all the flavor of traditional sauce.

1 tablespoon avocado oil or canola oil

2 pounds 90 percent lean ground turkey

½ onion, chopped

3 garlic cloves, minced

1 (24-ounce) can crushed tomatoes

1 cup low-sodium beef broth

3 tablespoons Italian seasoning

Salt and black pepper to taste

12 ounces whole-wheat spaghetti (¾ package)

1. In a large saucepan over medium-high heat, heat the oil until shimmering. Add the turkey and break it apart into small pieces with a spatula. Cook for approximately 5 minutes, or until the turkey is browned.

2. Add the onions and garlic to the pan and cook for another 2 to 3 minutes, until the onions turn translucent. Stir in the crushed tomatoes, beef broth, Italian seasoning, salt, and pepper.

3. Cook until the sauce begins to boil, then reduce the heat to low and cover with a lid. Allow the sauce to simmer for 25 minutes, stirring occasionally.

4. While the sauce cooks, begin cooking the pasta. Add 4 cups of water to a large stockpot and bring to a boil over medium-high heat. Add the pasta and cook according to the box instructions. Drain the pasta.

5. To serve, top each serving with meat sauce.

Recipe Tips: To make this recipe vegetarian, use vegetable broth instead of beef broth, and replace turkey with tempeh cooked according to package instructions. To make this recipe vegan, also omit the Parmesan cheese. To make this recipe gluten-free, use gluten-free pasta and ensure your broth is free of gluten. To make this recipe Paleo, omit pasta and use double the amount of zucchini noodles.

Storage: Divide spaghetti servings straight into airtight containers to store in the fridge for up to four days. If you're looking to save on prep time in the future, double or triple the sauce recipe and freeze the extras. Sauce by itself can be frozen for up to 3 months.

Nutritional Information: Calories: 363, Total Fat: 12g, Saturated Fat: 3g, Protein: 27g, Carbohydrates: 36g, Fiber: 6g, Sodium: 234mg

Slow Cooker Turkey Chili with Sweet Potatoes

YIELD: Serves 8 (1-cup servings) **PREP TIME:** 15 minutes **COOK TIME:** 4 to 10 hours

Slow cooker chili is one of the easiest winter recipes to make when you want something hearty and delicious. The complex carbohydrates and fiber from the sweet potatoes and beans will keep you feeling pleasantly full for hours.

1 tablespoon avocado oil

1 pound 90 percent lean ground turkey

2 (12-ounce) cans diced tomatoes

1 packet low-sodium taco seasoning

½ tablespoon chili powder

Black pepper to taste

1 (15-ounce) can black beans, drained

1 (15-ounce) can pinto beans, drained

1 (15-ounce) can garbanzo beans, drained

2 (4-ounce) cans diced green chiles

1 small onion, chopped

4 medium sweet potatoes

1. In a large skillet over medium-high heat, heat the oil until shimmering. Add the turkey and break it apart into small ground pieces with a spatula. Cook for approximately 5 minutes, or until the turkey is browned.

2. While the turkey is cooking, add the diced tomatoes to a slow cooker. Stir in the taco seasoning, chili powder, and black pepper, then add in the beans, chiles, and onions and mix well.

3. Add the turkey to the slow cooker and mix into the other ingredients, ensuring that the turkey is adequately covered by the tomatoes and beans. Cook on low for 8 to 10 hours, or on high for 4 to 5 hours.

4. Meanwhile, cook the sweet potatoes. Poke multiple small holes into each potato with a fork. In a microwave, cook on high for 10 to 12 minutes. Allow the potatoes to cool in the microwave for 5 minutes before handling. Once the potatoes are cool enough to touch, peel the skin and chop the potatoes into 2-inch chunks. Set aside.

5. To serve, place ½ cup of the chopped sweet potatoes into each of the bottoms of 8 bowls and spoon 1 cup of chili over the potatoes.

Recipe Tip: No slow cooker? No problem. To make this dish without a slow cooker, cook the turkey meat in a large saucepan. Add all of the additional ingredients, except the sweet potatoes, to the saucepan once the turkey is browned. Place a lid on the pot and cook on medium-low for 30 minutes, stirring occasionally. Cook the sweet potatoes in the microwave according to the original recipe directions.

Storage: Keep the sweet potatoes and chili separate when storing. The chili on its own can stay in the fridge for up to 3 days or in the freezer up to 3 months.

Nutritional Information: Calories: 436, Total Fat: 12g, Saturated Fat: 3g, Protein: 31g, Carbohydrates: 51g, Fiber: 11g, Sodium: 527mg

Garlic-Cilantro Salsa Chicken

YIELD: Serves 8 (1-cup servings) **PREP TIME:** 10 minutes **COOK TIME:** 20 minutes

If you're looking for a no-fuss recipe, you've hit the jackpot here. This salsa chicken takes only minutes to prepare but tastes like you slaved away in the kitchen for hours. This salsa is packed with antioxidants and protein. Antioxidants help prevent stress-induced damage to the body, while the protein promotes increased lean muscle mass and satiety.

6 medium tomatoes, roughly chopped

2 cloves garlic

4 ounces green chile peppers, diced

⅓ cup cilantro leaves, packed

½ teaspoon black pepper

⅛ teaspoon salt

½ lime, juiced

2 pounds boneless, skinless chicken breasts

1. Into a food processer, add the tomatoes, garlic, chile peppers, cilantro, black pepper, salt, and lime juice and blend for 30 seconds, or until the salsa appears smooth.

2. In the bottom of a large stockpot, place chicken breasts. The breasts may overlap slightly, if necessary. Add water to the pot until there is approximately 1 inch of water covering the chicken. Heat on high until the water begins to boil and bubbles appear on the surface. Reduce the heat to low and allow the chicken to simmer for 12 to 15 minutes or until the chicken is cooked through.

3. Move the cooked chicken from the pot to a cutting board. With two forks, shred the chicken into small pieces and then add back to the pot. Stir in the salsa until chicken is evenly coated. Serve.

Recipe Tips: The salsa can be prepared ahead of time and stored in the freezer for an easy weeknight meal. Just defrost in the fridge the day before use. If you're tight on time, a 16-ounce jar of fresh salsa can be used in place of the homemade recipe. Serve this dish with brown rice or another starchy carbohydrate of choice.

Storage: This chicken will keep in the fridge for up to 3 days or in the freezer for up to 3 months.

Nutritional Information: Calories: 135, Total Fat: 3g, Saturated Fat: 1g, Protein: 24g, Carbohydrates: 5g, Fiber: 2g, Sodium: 281mg

Baked Salmon with Zesty Lemon-Garlic Sauce

YIELD: Serves 4 **PREP TIME:** 10 minutes **COOK TIME:** 30 minutes

Lemon and garlic flavor this dish, and salmon is the perfect protein to accompany vegetables, grains, or even a hearty salad. Salmon provides a boost of anti-inflammatory omega-3 fatty acids in each bite, making this dish the perfect pick for a busy athlete.

2 tablespoons olive oil

3 cloves garlic, minced

1 teaspoon black pepper

4 scallions, chopped

2 lemons, divided

2 (8-ounce) skin-on salmon fillets, patted dry

1. Preheat oven to 400°F.

2. In a medium skillet over medium-high heat, heat the oil until shimmering. Add the garlic and sauté for 2 to 3 minutes, until the garlic becomes aromatic and begins to brown. Remove from the heat and allow the oil and garlic to cool for approximately 5 minutes.

3. Transfer the oil and garlic to a small mixing bowl. Add in the black pepper, scallions, and juice of one lemon.

4. Place the salmon fillets skin-side down, each on a large piece of aluminum foil. Gently rub the fillets liberally with the oil mixture using a basting or pastry brush. Slice the remaining lemon and arrange lemon slices on top of the fillets.

5. Fold the aluminum foil around each fish until it is completely sealed, making packets.

6. Place the foil packets on a baking sheet and place in the oven. Cook for 20 minutes, or until the fish flakes easily with a fork. Serve.

Recipe Tip: Serve the fish with broccoli and brown rice or over salad.

Storage: If storing, wrap the fish directly in foil and keep refrigerated for up to 3 days. To reheat, place foil with fish in a toaster oven or conventional oven and heat on low for 5 minutes, or until the fish is heated through.

Nutritional Information: Calories: 210, Total Fat: 12g, Saturated Fat: 3g, Protein: 23g, Carbohydrates: 8g, Fiber: 3g, Sodium: 175mg

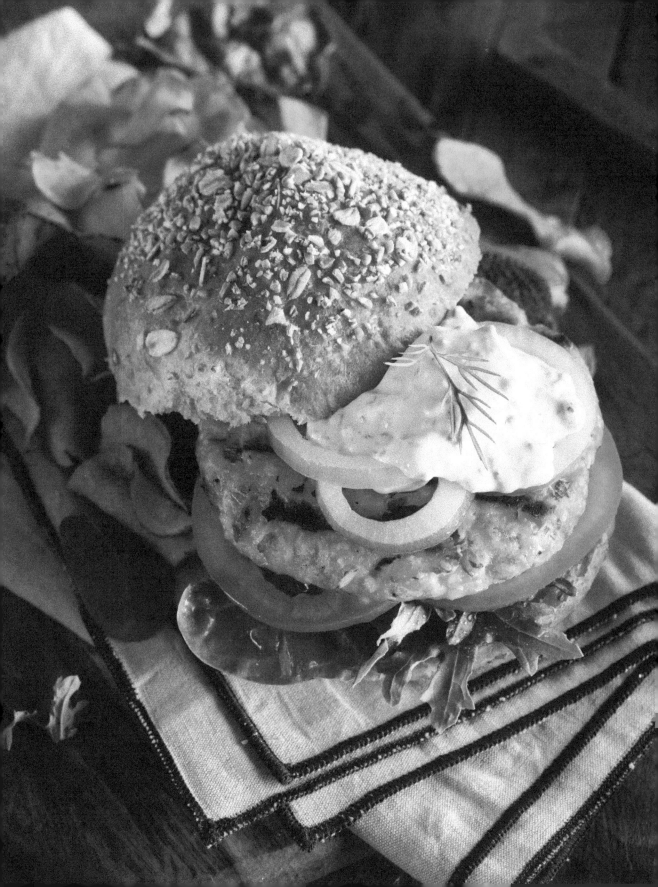

CHAPTER THIRTEEN

GAME DAY RECIPES

GAME DAY IS THE PERFECT TIME to focus on quick-digesting carbohydrates in order to keep your body fueled all day long during those intense competitions. The type of meal you choose to eat should be based on when your competition is. If you have any early-morning game and have only an hour or two to eat before stepping onto the field, opt for choices like smoothies, oatmeal, or French toast that are easy to digest. If your competition isn't until the afternoon or evening, or you have several hours to eat your next meal prior to performing, more balanced dishes such as sandwiches and wraps are easy to make ahead and eat on the go. By preparing ahead and having game day foods ready, you'll be fueled for success all day long.

Apple Pie Breakfast Smoothie

YIELD: Serves 1 **PREP TIME:** 5 minutes

This apple pie smoothie is so rich, it will leave you wondering if it's really good for you. The oats and Greek yogurt make this recipe thick and creamy, while providing a balance of carbohydrates and protein for your morning meal. With only 7 ingredients, this smoothie can be whipped up in just a few minutes and easily taken on the go.

1 large apple, core removed and chopped

½ banana, chopped

1 (5-ounce) container low-fat vanilla Greek yogurt

¼ cup old-fashioned oats

1 tablespoon honey

2 teaspoons apple pie spice

1 cup ice

1. Into a blender, put the apple, banana, yogurt, oats, honey, apple pie spice, and ice and blend until smooth.

2. Pour into a glass and serve immediately.

Recipe Tips: To make this dish gluten-free, be sure to purchase oats that have the GF label, as many are made on shared equipment with gluten-containing items. To make this recipe vegan, replace the honey with agave or maple syrup and use a plant-based Greek-style yogurt. Trouble finding apple pie spice? Substitute with 1 teaspoon of cinnamon.

Storage: This recipe is best consumed fresh. Smoothies can be left in the fridge for up to an hour before the ingredients begin to separate.

Nutritional Information: Calories: 452, Total Fat: 6g, Saturated Fat: 3g, Protein: 21g, Carbohydrates: 85g, Fiber: 11g, Sodium: 74mg

French Toast Bake

YIELD: Serves 3 (4 French toast halves per serving)
PREP TIME: 10 minutes **COOK TIME:** 30 minutes

What sounds better than a warm piece of French toast first thing in the morning? A French toast recipe that doesn't need you slaving over a skillet. This oven recipe will give you traditional, fluffy, and lightly sweetened French toast that will provide you with the carbohydrates and energy needed to start your day right.

4 large eggs

2 teaspoons cinnamon

1 teaspoon vanilla extract

1 cup low-fat milk

6 slices whole-wheat bread, cut in half

¼ cup honey or maple syrup

2 bananas, sliced

1. Preheat oven to 350°F.

2. In a medium mixing bowl, whisk together the eggs, cinnamon, vanilla extract, and milk. Pour the mixture into a 9-by-12-inch baking dish. Add in the bread slices and turn them until the bread is coated evenly on both sides. Arrange the slices so that they are not overlapping in the baking dish and let the pieces soak in the mixture for 5 minutes.

3. Place the dish in the oven and cook for 20 minutes. Remove from the oven and carefully drizzle honey or maple syrup over the bread. Top with banana slices. Place the dish back in the oven and cook for 10 more minutes. Serve.

Recipe Tips: To make this dish gluten-free, substitute gluten-free bread. To make this dish dairy-free, substitute the milk with unsweetened almond milk.

Storage: This dish can be made ahead and kept in the fridge without the honey or banana for up to 3 days. Add banana or honey immediately before serving.

Nutritional Information: Calories: 474, Total Fat: 10g, Saturated Fat: 3g, Protein: 20g, Carbohydrates: 83g, Fiber: 7g, Sodium: 407mg

Blueberry-Banana Oatmeal Squares

YIELD: Serves 8 **PREP TIME:** 10 minutes **COOK TIME:** 45 minutes

Baked oatmeal is one of the easiest ways to batch-cook a delicious and hearty breakfast for the week. Keep your oatmeal squares in the fridge for a quick and easy breakfast or pack them for a handheld pre-workout snack. Either way, this recipe is sure to satisfy your sweet tooth.

2 cups old-fashioned oats

2 teaspoons cinnamon

1 teaspoon baking powder

½ teaspoon salt

1½ cups low-fat milk

¼ cup honey

2 large eggs

1 teaspoon vanilla extract

1 cup blueberries, divided

1 tablespoon butter or coconut oil

1 large banana, sliced

4 cups nonfat plain Greek yogurt

1. Preheat oven to 375°F.

2. In a medium mixing bowl, combine the oats, cinnamon, baking powder, and salt and whisk until well combined. In a separate medium mixing bowl, whisk together the milk, honey, eggs, and vanilla extract. Add the dry ingredients into the wet mixture and whisk until combined. Carefully fold in half of the blueberries.

3. Grease a 9-inch baking pan with either butter or oil. Arrange the banana slices on the bottom of the pan, then top with the oatmeal mixture.

4. Sprinkle the remaining blueberries over the top of the mixture and bake for 40 to 45 minutes, or until the top of the oatmeal is golden brown and a fork comes out clean.

5. Cut into 8 squares and serve each with ½ cup of the yogurt.

Recipe Tip: To make this dish gluten-free, purchase oats with a GF label.

Storage: Keep these bars in the fridge for 4 days or in the freezer for up to 3 months.

Nutritional Information: Calories: 245, Total Fat: 5g, Saturated Fat: 2g, Protein: 18g, Carbohydrates: 36g, Fiber: 3g, Sodium: 306mg

Chicken Salad Sandwich

YIELD: Serves 2 **PREP TIME:** 5 to 10 minutes

Nothing beats Thanksgiving with the family, but this Thanksgiving-inspired Chicken Salad Sandwich does come close. The combination of chicken, cranberries, and parsley will make you feel like you're sitting at the dinner table with your family and friends on that late November night. Dried cranberries have a number of health benefits for athletes, including a high antioxidant profile, immune-boosting properties, and the ability to help aid in digestion.

⅛ cup low-fat mayonnaise

⅛ teaspoon salt

¼ teaspoon black pepper

½ tablespoon dried
  parsley flakes

8 ounces chicken breast,
  cooked and cut into
  1-inch cubes

¼ cup dried cranberries

½ celery stalk, diced

⅛ cup sliced almonds

⅛ cup diced red onion

4 slices whole-wheat bread

1. In a large bowl, mix together the mayonnaise, salt, pepper, and parsley. Add in the chicken, dried cranberries, celery, almonds, and onions. Mix until well combined and all ingredients are coated.

2. Divide the mixture evenly onto the four slices of bread and serve open-faced.

Recipe Tips: No almonds in the pantry? Use pecans or walnut halves instead. No cooked chicken on hand? Swap out chicken breast for skinless rotisserie chicken to save on cooking and prep time.

Storage: Store chicken salad in the fridge for up to 3 days.

Nutritional Information: Calories: 411, Total Fat: 9g, Saturated Fat: 1g, Protein: 33g, Carbohydrates: 57g, Fiber: 9g, Sodium: 846mg

Avocado Egg Salad

YIELD: Serves 2 (1/2-cup servings) **PREP TIME:** 5 minutes **COOK TIME:** 15 minutes

Avocado provides all of the creaminess that's in traditional egg salad, but with a powerful nutrient boost of vitamins and omega-3 fatty acids that aren't typically found in mayo-based egg salad. The simple addition of dill and parsley makes this salad or sandwich filling a flavor powerhouse.

4 large eggs	**½ tablespoon dried dill**	**½ teaspoon salt**
1 avocado	**½ tablespoon dried parsley**	**1 teaspoon black pepper**

1. Place the eggs into a medium saucepan and fill with water until the eggs are fully submerged. Bring the water to a boil, then turn the burner off, cover the pot with a lid, and allow it to sit for approximately 10 minutes. Once the eggs are cool enough to handle, run under cold water and peel the shells. Set aside.

2. In a medium bowl, mash the avocado with a potato masher or metal spoon until most of the large lumps have been removed. Add the eggs to the bowl and mash with a fork until well blended.

3. Add the dill, parsley, salt, and pepper to the bowl and mix until well combined. Serve.

Recipe Tips: If your avocados are going bad faster than you can use them, as soon as the skin begins turning brown and the avocados are slightly soft to the touch, toss them into the fridge to prolong their life (and deliciousness). Serve this salad on whole-wheat bread, a lettuce wrap, or over salad with a side of fruit.

Storage: Due to how fast avocados brown, this recipe is best eaten fresh.

Nutritional Information: Calories: 294, Total Fat: 23g, Saturated Fat: 5g, Protein: 15g, Carbohydrates: 10g, Fiber: 6g, Sodium: 734mg

Turkey and Avocado BLT Mini-Wraps

YIELD: Serves 2 PREP TIME: 20 minutes

Long Island has amazing delis that make some of the best cold-cut sandwiches in the country. These turkey and avocado BLT mini-wraps are a makeover of one of my favorite deli sandwiches, and they only take a few minutes to put together.

2 (10-inch) whole-wheat tortillas

4 ounces low-sodium turkey breast deli meat (4 to 6 slices)

2 slices center-cut bacon or turkey bacon, cooked according to package instructions

1 cup lettuce, shredded

½ small avocado, sliced

1 small tomato, sliced

2 cups baby carrots

1. Lay the tortillas flat on parchment paper or a cutting board. Top each with half of the turkey, 1 slice of the bacon, ½ cup of the lettuce, half of the sliced avocado, and half of the sliced tomato. Firmly roll the tortilla up and slice in half with a knife.

2. Serve each wrap (2 pieces) with 1 cup baby carrots

Recipe Tips: If you want to change this wrap up, swap out the turkey deli meat for any other low-sodium choice you have on hand. If you're making these in advance, omit the avocado or replace with low-fat mayonnaise to avoid browning.

Nutritional Information: Calories: 370, Total Fat: 13g, Saturated Fat: 3g, Protein: 20g, Carbohydrates: 44g, Fiber: 8g, Sodium: 1,024mg

Sheet Pan Rosemary Chicken and Vegetables

YIELD: Serves 4 PREP TIME: 10 minutes COOK TIME: 32 minutes

Rosemary is an aromatic herb that gives this dish its savory taste. Sheet pan recipes are the perfect way to do minimal prep work and still have a tasty meal ready to eat. The mix of starchy and non-starchy carbohydrates in this dish provides an array of different vitamins, minerals, complex carbohydrates, and fiber in just one meal.

1 tablespoon olive oil

2 tablespoons fresh rosemary (or 2 teaspoons dried rosemary)

1 tablespoon dried thyme

2 garlic cloves, minced

½ teaspoon salt

1 teaspoon black pepper

1 pound boneless, skinless chicken thighs or breast meat

2 pounds sweet potatoes, quartered

2 cups asparagus, ends removed

1. Preheat oven to 400°F.

2. Line a sheet pan with aluminum foil and then parchment paper. Set aside.

3. In a large bowl, combine the oil, rosemary, thyme, garlic, salt, and pepper. Add the chicken and potatoes, and toss to coat evenly.

4. Place the chicken and potatoes on the sheet pan and bake for 20 minutes.

5. Add the asparagus to the bowl containing the herb mixture and toss to coat evenly. Place the asparagus on top of the chicken and potatoes, and cook for an additional 12 minutes.

6. Serve immediately.

Recipe Tips: To make this dish vegetarian, replace the chicken with tofu or 2 cups of additional sweet potato or asparagus. Want to change the recipe up or don't have the right vegetables on hand? Swap the sweet potatoes out for white potatoes or peeled, chopped butternut squash. The asparagus can be swapped for green beans or broccoli. This recipe can also be pre-portioned and put into food containers for quick lunches or dinners throughout the week.

Storage: Keep this dish in the fridge for up to 4 days.

Nutritional Information: Calories: 358, Total Fat: 7g, Saturated Fat: 1g, Protein: 28g, Carbohydrates: 50g, Fiber: 9g, Sodium: 598mg

Simple Chicken Pasta

YIELD: Serves 2 **PREP TIME:** 5 minutes **COOK TIME:** 10 minutes

Don't be fooled by the simple ingredient list. This chicken pasta recipe has the perfect balance of complex carbohydrates, protein, and fat to keep your body fueled and your taste buds satisfied.

4 ounces whole-wheat penne pasta

½ tablespoon avocado oil or butter

1 cup broccoli florets

6 ounces cooked chicken breast, diced

½ cup peas, drained

2 teaspoons garlic powder

¼ teaspoon salt

½ teaspoon black pepper

¼ cup Parmesan cheese

1. Add 4 cups of water to a large stockpot and bring to a boil over high heat. Add the pasta and cook according to package directions, stirring occasionally.

2. While the pasta cooks, prepare the broccoli. In a medium sauté pan over medium-high heat, heat the oil or butter. Add the broccoli and sauté for 5 minutes, or until cooked through. Set aside.

3. Drain the pasta and add to a large mixing bowl. Add the broccoli, chicken, peas, garlic powder, salt, and pepper. Stir well to combine and let cool for 5 minutes.

4. Serve each portion with half of the Parmesan cheese sprinkled on top.

Recipe Tip: To make this dish dairy-free, omit the Parmesan cheese and toss the pasta with 1 tablespoon olive oil. To make this gluten-free, cook with GF pasta.

Storage: You can store this dish in the fridge for up to 3 days.

Nutritional Information: Calories: 436, Total Fat: 11g, Saturated Fat: 4g, Protein: 36g, Carbohydrates: 44g, Fiber: 9g, Sodium: 630mg

Salmon Burgers with Baked Sweet Potatoes

YIELD: Serves 2 **PREP TIME:** 15 minutes **COOK TIME:** 25 minutes

Looking to pack as much nutrition as possible into a burger patty? Look no further than these salmon burgers. Full of vitamin D, omega-3 fatty acids, B12, and protein, this meal is an excellent way to fuel your recovery as much as your stomach.

2 medium sweet potatoes

1 teaspoon olive oil cooking spray

¼ teaspoon salt, divided

½ teaspoon black pepper, divided

1 teaspoon paprika

2 (4-ounce) salmon burger patties, fresh or frozen

2 teaspoons avocado oil or butter

2 whole-wheat hamburger buns

½ cup arugula

tartar sauce (optional)

1. Preheat oven to 375°F.

2. Peel the sweet potatoes and cut into long, quarter-inch thick wedges. Place the potato wedges in a medium bowl and spray with the cooking spray, turning to coat.

3. Line a baking sheet with parchment paper. Add the potatoes and sprinkle with half of the salt and pepper, as well as all the paprika. Bake for 20 to 25 minutes, or until the wedges look golden brown, turning the wedges halfway through the cooking time.

4. While the potato wedges are cooking, prepare the salmon patties. Sprinkle the patties with the remaining salt and pepper. In a large skillet over medium heat, heat the oil or butter. Add the patties and cook approximately 5 minutes per side (or 8 minutes per side if using frozen patties), until a meat thermometer inserted into the center reaches an internal temperature of 145°F.

5. Arrange the buns on plates. Place a salmon burger on each bun and top with arugula and the tartar sauce, if using. Serve immediately with sweet potato wedges.

Salmon Burgers with Baked Sweet Potatoes CONTINUED

Recipe Tips: Salmon patties are delicious but may not always be readily available. Feel free to swap out with ground turkey, chicken, or beef burgers instead. If you're in a time crunch, pre-packaged potato wedges that have minimal added oil or processed ingredients on the food label can be swapped in instead.

Nutritional Information: Calories: 505, Total Fat: 18g, Saturated Fat: 2g, Protein: 30g, Carbohydrates: 57g, Fiber: 8g, Sodium: 850mg

Baked Veggie Mac 'n' Cheese

YIELD: Serves 8 (1-cup servings) **PREP TIME:** 20 minutes **COOK TIME:** 30 minutes

Even athletes need comfort food once in a while. This baked veggie mac 'n' cheese packs all the flavor of traditional mac, but has a big nutrient boost from broccoli and carrots. This is the perfect dish to make ahead and eat throughout the week or on game day to get a boost of carbohydrates.

1½ cups whole-grain elbow macaroni

3 cups broccoli florets

3 carrots, diced small

1 tablespoon butter or avocado oil

2 tbsp all-purpose flour

1 cup low-sodium chicken broth

1 cup low-fat milk

2 cups shredded low-fat cheddar cheese

½ teaspoon black pepper

¼ teaspoon salt

½ teaspoon paprika

1. Preheat oven to 350°F.

2. Add 4 cups of water to a large stockpot and bring to a boil over high heat. Add the elbow macaroni and cook according to package instructions. When the macaroni has 5 to 6 minutes left, add in the broccoli and carrots. Finish cooking, then drain the pasta and vegetables, and transfer to a 13-by-9-inch baking dish. Set aside.

3. While the macaroni is cooking, in a medium saucepan over medium heat, heat the butter or oil. Add the flour and gradually stir in the chicken broth and milk, whisking frequently. Bring the mixture to a boil and let cook for 3 minutes, or until the liquid begins to thicken. Add in the cheese, pepper, and salt.

4. Gently pour the cheese sauce into the baking dish and stir to mix until the pasta has been evenly coated. Sprinkle paprika over the mixture.

5. Place into the oven and cook for 20 minutes or until the macaroni begins to brown.

Recipe Tip: Not a fan of broccoli or carrots? Swap them out with zucchini, yellow squash, or peas instead. The final dish with still taste great and be packed with extra vitamins or minerals.

Storage: This recipe will keep well in the fridge for up to 5 days. Just cover with foil and place the whole baking dish directly in the refrigerator once cool.

Nutritional Information: Calories: 213, Total Fat: 7g, Saturated Fat: 4g, Protein: 12g, Carbohydrates: 22g, Fiber: 3g, Sodium: 360mg

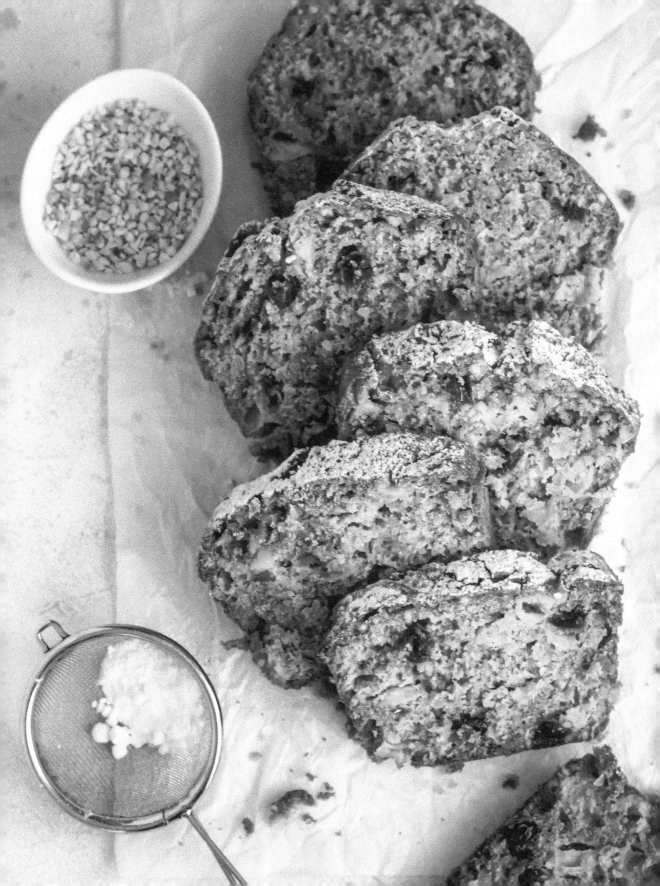

CHAPTER FOURTEEN

POSTGAME AND RECOVERY DAY RECIPES

ONCE A COMPETITION IS OVER, one of the most important things an athlete can do is rest and recover so that they're at 100 percent come their next training day or practice. For recovery meals, the focus is on replenishing muscle glycogen and energy stores with carbohydrates, repairing muscle tissue with protein, getting in a moderate amount of fat to balance out calories, and consuming the proper vitamins, minerals, and fluids to stay hydrated and to strengthen your immune system. Meals during a recovery day or postgame should still be balanced and spread throughout the day. Skip any pre- and post-workout snacks you typically consume if you're not training on your recovery day, and instead focus on balanced meals.

Overnight Blueberry-Banana Oatmeal

YIELD: Serves 1 **PREP TIME:** 5 to 10 minutes

This overnight oatmeal recipe is the perfect make-ahead breakfast for a busy athlete. This oatmeal is packed with vitamin C and antioxidants, and is a plant-based source of omega-3 fatty acids. If you're looking for a quick grab-and-go breakfast in the morning, this oatmeal is for you.

1 cup old-fashioned oats

1 teaspoon ground cinnamon

½ cup blueberries

½ cup strawberries, sliced

1 cup low-fat milk

2 tablespoons honey

¼ cup nonfat plain Greek yogurt

⅛ cup walnuts, chopped

1. In a mason jar or airtight container, mix the oats and cinnamon. Without mixing further, layer the blueberries and strawberries. Add the milk, honey, and yogurt. Cover with a lid or plastic wrap and refrigerate overnight.

2. When ready to serve, shake the jar or stir to combine. Add the walnuts right before serving.

Recipe Tip: This recipe is extremely versatile. Swap out the berries and walnuts with your favorite fruit and nut of choice. Some great flavor combinations include apples and walnuts, bananas and walnuts, or sliced strawberries and sliced almonds.

Storage: The pre-shaken mixture can be stored in the fridge for up to 48 hours.

Nutritional Information: Calories: 727, Total Fat: 19g, Saturated Fat: 2g, Protein: 27g, Carbohydrates: 122g, Fiber: 14g, Sodium: 157mg

Tofu Scramble

YIELD: Serves 2 **PREP TIME:** 5 minutes **COOK TIME:** 15 minutes

This vegetarian breakfast dish is full of plant-based protein to keep you full all morning. The tofu used as the base of this dish is high in a number of vitamins and minerals, including iron, calcium, magnesium, copper, and B1, all of which help provide balanced energy throughout the day and improve both heart health and immune function.

8 ounces firm or extra-firm tofu	½ cup diced red pepper	¼ teaspoon turmeric
	½ cup diced onion	¼ teaspoon black pepper
1 tablespoon avocado oil	¼ cup scallions, thinly sliced	¼ teaspoon salt

1. Chop the tofu into small pieces and use a fork to crumble.
2. In a medium sauté pan over medium-high heat, heat the oil. Add the peppers and onions and cook for 5 minutes, stirring frequently. Add the tofu, scallions, turmeric, pepper, and salt. Mix well. Cook the scramble for 10 minutes, stirring occasionally.
3. Serve.

Recipe Tips: If you're not a fan of peppers and onions, replace them with another vegetable of choice. A few good flavor options include tomatoes, potatoes, broccoli, or grated zucchini. Serve this dish with fruit or whole-wheat bread.

Storage: This scramble can be stored in the fridge for up to 4 days.

Nutritional Information: Calories: 203, Total Fat: 13g, Saturated Fat: 2g, Protein: 13g, Carbohydrates: 11g, Fiber: 3g, Sodium: 328mg

Banana-Walnut Bread

YIELD: Serves 8 **PREP TIME:** 10 minutes **COOK TIME:** 45 minutes

This banana-walnut bread is extremely moist and lightly sweetened to perfection. The recipe is one we've been making in my family for years and will certainly not disappoint. The bread is rich in quick-digesting carbohydrates that will provide immediate energy right before a big tournament or game.

4 bananas

1 large egg

¼ cup low-fat milk

¼ cup honey

2 tablespoons applesauce

½ teaspoon salt

1 teaspoon baking soda

½ teaspoon baking powder

¾ cup whole-wheat flour

¾ cup white flour

¼ cup walnut halves

1 tablespoon canola oil
  or butter

1. Preheat oven to 350°F.

2. In a large mixing bowl, mash the bananas with a fork until all large lumps have been removed. Add in the egg, milk, honey, and applesauce and mix well.

3. In a separate mixing bowl, combine the salt, baking soda, baking powder, and flours. Mix well, then add to the banana mixture. Gently fold the walnut halves into the batter with a rubber spatula.

4. Grease a medium-size loaf pan with canola oil or butter. Add the batter to the loaf pan and bake for 45 minutes or until a toothpick comes out clean.

Recipe Tips: No applesauce? Swap it out with 2 tablespoons of canola oil instead. Since this bread is the perfect grab-and-go option for a busy schedule, preparing it ahead of time and wrapping pieces individually in plastic wrap or storing in a container in the fridge makes it even easier to pick up. This bread can stay in a lunch box or backpack without refrigeration if it's being eaten the same day.

Storage: This bread has minimal preservatives and will go bad if left at room temperature. Store in the fridge for 3 days or in the freezer for up to 3 months.

Nutritional Information: Calories: 212, Total Fat: 5g, Saturated Fat: 1g, Protein: 5g, Carbohydrates: 40g, Fiber: 4g, Sodium: 347mg

Protein-Packed Fruity Smoothie

YIELD: Serves 2 **PREP TIME:** 5 minutes

Smoothies are a great all-in-one meal for on the go. This recipe is packed with vitamins C and K and plant-based omega-3 fatty acids. Fresh or frozen fruit can be used for this tasty recipe.

½ cup strawberries

½ cup blueberries

½ large banana

½ cup low-fat vanilla
Greek yogurt

8 ounces low-fat milk

1 tablespoon flaxseed

1 cup ice

Into a blender, add the strawberries, blueberries, banana, yogurt, milk, flaxseed, and ice and blend until smooth. Serve immediately.

Recipe Tip: Looking to get more protein in during the day? Add a scoop of whey protein isolate or an additional half cup of Greek yogurt for a boost.

Storage: This smoothie is best consumed fresh but can be stored in the fridge for up to an hour before the ingredients begin to separate.

Nutritional Information: Calories: 177, Total Fat: 5g, Saturated Fat: 2g, Protein: 11g, Carbohydrates: 25g, Fiber: 4g, Sodium: 91mg

Chicken Tortilla Soup

YIELD: Serves 6 (1½-cup servings)
PREP TIME: 10 minutes **COOK TIME:** 20 minutes

This spicy and hearty soup is chock-full of complex carbohydrates and protein, making it the perfect choice for a recovery meal. The fiber, B vitamins, and phytonutrient profile of black beans also helps support heart health while keeping the body fueled. The tortilla chips are the secret ingredient to making this soup thick and crunchy.

3 cups whole-wheat tortilla chips, divided

1 tablespoon avocado or canola oil

4 cups low-sodium chicken broth

1 (28-ounce) can low-sodium pureéd tomatoes

2 tablespoons tomato paste

½ tablespoon garlic powder

1 teaspoon chili powder

½ teaspoon cumin

1½ pounds skinless rotisserie chicken or cooked chicken breast, cut into 1-inch cubes or shredded

1 (15-ounce) can black beans, drained and rinsed

Salt and pepper to taste

1. Place half of the tortilla chips into a bowl. Gently crush the chips into small pieces and set aside.

2. In a large saucepan over medium-high heat, heat the oil. Add in the chicken broth, tomatoes, tomato paste, garlic powder, chili powder, and cumin. Once the liquid comes to a boil, add in the chicken and beans and mix well. Reduce the heat and bring the soup to a simmer. Cook for 10 minutes.

3. Mix in the crushed tortilla chips and cook for another 10 minutes. Season with salt and pepper.

4. Ladle 1½ cups of soup into a bowl, garnishing each with the remaining tortilla chips before serving.

Recipe Tip: Don't have all the spices needed on hand? Swap out the cumin, chili powder, garlic, salt, and pepper with 2 tablespoons of low-sodium taco seasoning instead.

Storage: Store in the fridge for up to 3 days. To save time during the week, put servings into individual containers and refrigerate for easy access. To freeze this recipe, omit the tortilla chips during the cooking process and add as a garnish to your bowl after reheating.

Nutritional Information: Calories: 370, Total Fat: 6g, Saturated Fat: 1g, Protein: 34g, Carbohydrates: 26g, Fiber: 4g, Sodium: 179mg

Teriyaki Chicken Stir-Fry

YIELD: Serves 6 (1½-cup servings)
PREP TIME: 10 minutes **COOK TIME:** 15 minutes

Chicken teriyaki was a favorite of mine as a kid. Whenever we were fortunate enough to go to a Japanese restaurant, this was my go-to order. Luckily, this homemade version hits the spot just as well. Ginger gives this dish an authentic flavor while also providing anti-inflammatory benefits and may even help reduce muscle soreness.

4 tablespoons low-sodium
  soy sauce
1 tablespoon honey
1 teaspoon dried ginger
  or 1 tablespoon fresh
  grated ginger

1 tablespoon
  all-purpose flour
1½ tablespoons avocado or
  canola oil, divided
2 cloves garlic, minced

1½ pounds chicken breast,
  cut into ½-inch cubes
¼ teaspoon salt
½ teaspoon black pepper
1½ cups broccoli florets

1. In a bowl, combine the soy sauce, honey, ginger, and flour. Set aside.

2. In a large non-stick sauté pan or wok over medium-high heat, heat 2 teaspoons of the oil. Add the garlic and cook for 1 to 2 minutes, until golden brown. Remove from the pan and set aside.

3. Add 1 teaspoon of oil to the same pan. Sprinkle the chicken with salt and pepper and add to the pan. Cook for 5 to 6 minutes, or until the chicken is fully cooked.

4. While chicken cooks, make the broccoli. In a large skillet over medium-high heat, heat ½ tablespoon of the oil. Add the broccoli and sauté for 4 to 5 minutes.

5. Add the chicken to the skillet with the broccoli and then add the sauce and garlic. Sauté for 1 minute. Serve.

Recipe Tips: Teriyaki is an easy dish to get creative with. Swap out the chicken for beef, pork, salmon, or shrimp to change it up. If you're not a fan of broccoli, use a different veggie instead, such as green beans, asparagus, or even carrots. Serve with brown rice.

Storage: Place in a container and store in refrigerator for up to 3 days.

Nutritional Information: Calories: 174, Total Fat: 6g, Saturated Fat: 1g, Protein: 24g, Carbohydrates: 6g, Fiber: 1g, Sodium: 666mg

Fiesta Chicken Tacos

YIELD: Serves 2 **PREP TIME:** 10 minutes **COOK TIME:** 20 minutes

Tacos are no longer reserved just for Tuesdays. These chicken tacos have all the flavor of traditional tacos without all of the fat that usually comes with ground beef. This protein-packed dish is sure to satisfy your taco cravings as it gives you a boost of protein.

½ tablespoon avocado or canola oil

8 ounces boneless skinless chicken breast

½ packet of low-sodium taco seasoning

4 (6-inch) whole-wheat tortillas

1 medium tomato, diced

½ cup onion, finely diced

1 cup lettuce or kale, shredded

¼ cup low-sodium shredded cheddar cheese

1. In a large skillet over medium-high heat, heat the oil. Rub the chicken with taco seasoning until well coated, then add to the skillet. Cook for 6 to 7 minutes per side, until fully cooked through. Remove from the heat and let cool for 5 minutes. Once the chicken is cool enough to handle, cut into 1-inch-thick cubes.

2. Assemble the tacos: Onto each tortilla, evenly divide the chicken, tomatoes, onions, lettuce, and cheese. Serve.

Recipe Tips: In a rush or just don't feel like chopping up veggies? Swap out the tomato and onion for a cup of low-sodium store-bought pico de gallo or salsa instead. The tacos are also good with avocado slices and a dollop of nonfat Greek yogurt.

Nutritional Information: Calories: 500, Total Fat: 17g, Saturated Fat: 6g, Protein: 35g, Carbohydrates: 52g, Fiber: 6g, Sodium: 1,169mg

Chicken Tenders with Carrot Fries

YIELD: Serves 4 **PREP TIME:** 15 minutes **COOK TIME:** 16 minutes

These chicken tenders have all of the flavor and crunch of their traditional frozen or fast-food counterparts without all of the oil. The combination of whole-wheat bread crumbs and Japanese panko is the secret to making these tenders perfect. Pair them with some crispy carrot fries, and you've got yourself the perfect finger-food meal.

3 tablespoons whole-wheat bread crumbs

3 tablespoons panko bread crumbs

1 tablespoon Italian seasoning

1 teaspoon onion powder

2 teaspoons paprika

6 tablespoons grated Parmesan cheese, divided

1 large egg or 1 tablespoon olive oil

1 pound skinless chicken breast, cut into 3-inch strips

4 medium carrots

Olive oil cooking spray

¼ teaspoon salt

1 teaspoon black pepper

1. Preheat oven to 425°F.

2. Line a baking sheet with parchment paper.

3. In a small mixing bowl, combine the bread crumbs, panko, Italian seasoning, onion powder, paprika, and half of the cheese. In a separate bowl, beat the egg.

4. Using a fork or tongs, dip the chicken strips into the egg wash and then into the bread crumb mixture, ensuring that each piece is evenly coated. Place the chicken onto the baking sheet.

5. Slice the carrots in half length-wise, and then cut each piece in half lengthwise again to get thin strips. Place the carrots onto the baking sheet with the chicken.

6. Spray the chicken and carrots lightly with cooking spray, and season with salt and pepper. Bake the chicken and fries for approximately 16 minutes, or until chicken is cooked through, flipping both the carrots and chicken halfway through the cooking time. Sprinkle with the remaining cheese and serve.

Recipe Tips: To make this dish gluten-free, replace the flour and panko bread crumbs with 5½ tablespoons of almond flour and ½ tablespoon of coconut flour. To make this dish dairy-free, omit the Parmesan cheese or substitute ½ tablespoon of nutritional yeast.

Storage: The breading on these chicken strips will get spongy in the fridge, so this dish is best eaten fresh. To avoid prep time during the week, mix the ingredients for the breading in advance and store in an airtight container in the fridge for up to 48 hours.

Nutritional Information: Calories: 233, Total Fat: 6g, Saturated Fat: 2g, Protein: 30g, Carbohydrates: 16g, Fiber: 3g, Sodium: 534mg

Quinoa Burrito Bowls

YIELD: Serves 4 **PREP TIME:** 5 minutes **COOK TIME:** 30 minutes

Quinoa is a gluten-free grain that has double the protein of traditional rice and is a good source of fiber. These Quinoa Burrito Bowls will not only keep you fuller longer than a traditional rice bowl, but also are packed with extra iron, copper, and vitamin B6, which help with energy balance, focus, and strengthening the immune system.

1 tablespoon avocado or canola oil

1 pound 90 percent lean ground turkey

1 packet low-sodium taco seasoning

1 (16-ounce) can diced tomatoes

1 cup quinoa

1½ cups water

1 lime, juiced

¼ teaspoon salt

3 teaspoons dried cilantro, divided

2 cups shredded lettuce

1 medium avocado, sliced

1. In a large skillet over medium-high heat, heat the oil. Add the turkey and taco seasoning, gently breaking up the pieces with a spatula, and cook for 7 minutes, or until the turkey is browned. Add the diced tomatoes and cook for another 5 minutes until the turkey is cooked through. Remove from the heat and set aside.

2. While turkey is cooking, in a large saucepan over medium heat, place the quinoa and water, and bring to a boil. Once the water is boiling, reduce the heat to low and cook for 22 to 25 minutes, or until all liquid has been absorbed. Fluff with a fork and remove from the heat. Add in the lime juice, salt, and half of the cilantro and mix well. Set aside.

3. To prepare each bowl, place ¾ cup quinoa, ½ cup lettuce, and a quarter of the ground turkey in a bowl. Top with the avocado slices and remaining cilantro and serve immediately.

Recipe Tips: Quinoa can be swapped out for brown rice in these bowls. If you're looking to prep ahead, you can double or even triple the turkey meat and quinoa in this recipe and store in the freezer for up to 3 months.

Storage: Burrito bowls will stay good in the fridge for up to 3 days.

Nutritional Information: Calories: 489, Total Fat: 19g, Saturated Fat: 4g, Protein: 28g, Carbohydrates: 45g, Fiber: 7g, Sodium: 1,027mg

Turkey Shepherd's Pie

YIELD: Serves 4 **PREP TIME:** 15 minutes **COOK TIME:** 50 minutes

Traditional shepherd's pie can take hours to make, but this version was created with busy athletes in mind. Packed with protein and a variety of different vegetables and carbohydrates, this meal is sure to help replenish your glycogen stores the day after a strenuous competition.

3 tablespoons butter or avocado oil, divided

3 carrots, diced small

1 onion, diced small

1 pound 90 percent lean ground turkey

Salt and black pepper to taste

3 large russet potatoes

2 teaspoons garlic powder

2 tablespoons tomato paste

2 cups low-sodium beef broth

1 tablespoon Worcestershire sauce

1. Preheat oven to 400°F.

2. In a large saucepan over medium-high heat, heat 1 tablespoon of the butter or oil. Add the carrots and cook for 5 minutes, stirring frequently. Add the onions and cook for an additional 3 minutes. Set aside.

3. In a separate sauté pan over medium heat, heat 1 tablespoon of the butter or oil. Add the turkey, gently breaking up the pieces with a spatula. Season with salt and pepper, and cook for approximately 8 minutes, or until turkey is cooked through.

4. While the turkey is cooking, make the mashed potatoes. Carefully poke multiple holes in each potato with a fork and microwave on high for 10 to 12 minutes, or until the potatoes are soft. When the potatoes are cool enough to handle, peel and place them in a large mixing bowl. Add 1 tablespoon of butter or oil along with the garlic powder. With a potato masher or large fork, mash the potatoes until smooth.

5. Return the pan with the carrots and onions to medium heat and add the turkey, mixing thoroughly. Add the tomato paste, beef broth, and Worcestershire sauce. Let cook for an additional 5 minutes and remove from the heat.

6. Place the meat and vegetable mixture in a 13-by-9-inch baking dish. Evenly spread the mashed potatoes over the top and bake for 25 to 30 minutes, or until the potatoes begin to brown. Serve.

Nutritional Information: Calories: 506, Total Fat: 18g, Saturated Fat: 8g, Protein: 29g, Carbohydrates: 59g, Fiber: 8g, Sodium: 478mg

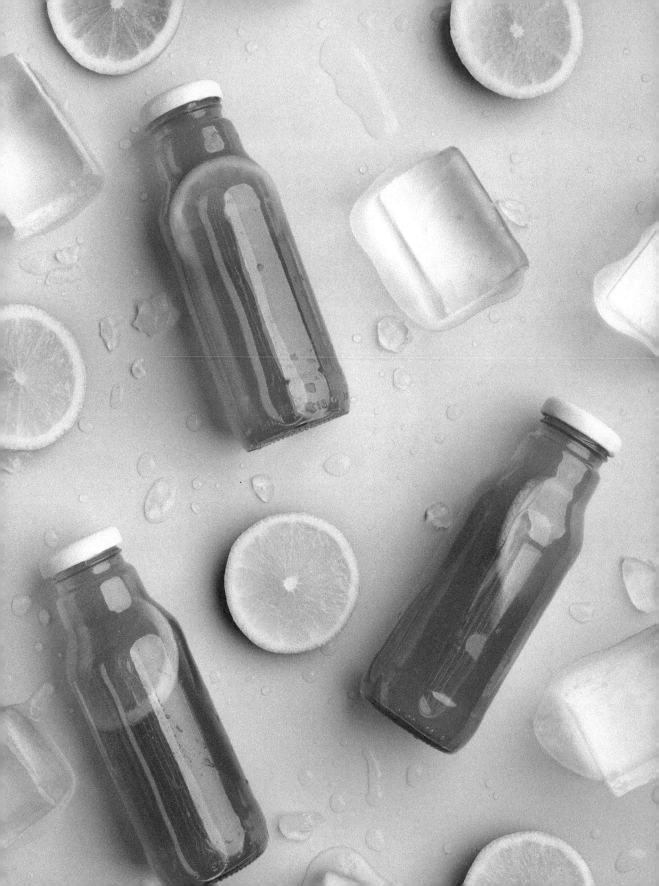

CHAPTER FIFTEEN

HOMEMADE SPORTS DRINK RECIPES

IF YOUR GAME DAY OR PRACTICE lasts longer than an hour, or if you train in extreme weather conditions, a sports drink may be necessary to adequately recover both your fluids and electrolytes. Choosing a homemade sports drink over a store-bought version means you get exactly what your body needs without the risk of consuming artificial flavors, sweeteners, or dyes. These sports drink recipes take just minutes to make and are extremely light, refreshing, and energizing.

Tropical Watermelon Sports Drink

YIELD: Serves 1 **PREP TIME:** 5 minutes

What could be more refreshing on a hot summer's day than watermelon? The combination of sweet coconut and watermelon in this drink will not only leave you refreshed, but will also pump up your glycogen and electrolyte levels so that you can play harder, longer.

6 ounces coconut water, unsweetened

4 ounces water

1 cup seedless chopped watermelon

dash salt

1. In a blender, add the coconut water, water, watermelon, and salt and blend in 10-second intervals until the drink is well mixed.

2. Serve immediately or keep chilled in the fridge or a cooler for up to 3 hours.

Storage: Need your sports drink to last longer? Place in a freezer-friendly bottle or container and put directly in the freezer after mixing. Take out of the freezer at least 5 to 6 hours before needed and shake well before drinking.

Nutritional Information: Calories: 81, Total Fat: <1g, Saturated Fat: 0g, Protein: 1g, Carbohydrates: 20g, Fiber: 1g, Sodium: 60mg

Lemon and Citrus Sports Drink

YIELD: Serves 1 **PREP TIME:** 5 minutes **COOK TIME:** 1 minute

If you're looking for a refreshing, tangy beverage to have with you on the field, then you're in the right place. The combination of citrus and lemon will leave you feeling alert and invigorated while providing a boost of vitamin C and antioxidants.

14 ounces water, divided
$\frac{1}{10}$ teaspoon salt

¼ lemon, juiced

6 ounces orange juice, pulp-free

1. In a microwave, in a large microwave-safe cup or bowl, heat ½ cup of water for 30 seconds. Add the salt and stir until dissolved.

2. Add the remaining 6 ounces of water, lemon juice, and orange juice. Serve immediately or pour into a container and chill for up to 1 day.

Storage: Need your sports drink to last longer? Place in a freezer-friendly bottle or container and put directly in the freezer after mixing. Take out of the freezer at least 4 to 5 hours before needed and shake well before drinking.

Nutritional Information: Calories: 85, Total Fat: 1g, Saturated Fat: <1g, Protein: 2g, Carbohydrates: 20g, Fiber: <1g, Sodium: 24mg

Strawberry and Lime Sports Drink

YIELD: Serves 1 **PREP TIME:** 5 minutes **COOK TIME:** 1 minute

Want to quench your thirst while replenishing your electrolytes, fluids, and glycogen? This Strawberry and Lime Sports Drink is perfect. With a hint of sweetness from honey and a refreshing flavor from strawberries, this is hands-down one of my favorite go-to recipes when I need a pick-me-up during training.

20 ounces water, divided

$\frac{1}{10}$ teaspoon salt

4 strawberries, halved lengthwise with tops removed

¼ lime, juiced

3 tablespoons honey

1. In a microwave, in a large microwave-safe cup or bowl, heat ½ cup of water for 30 seconds. Add the salt and stir until dissolved.

2. Add the remaining 2 cups water, strawberries, lime juice, and honey. Serve immediately or pour into a container and chill up to 24 hours.

Storage: Need your sports drink to last longer? Place in a freezer-friendly bottle or container and put directly in the freezer after mixing. Take out of the freezer at least 4 to 5 hours before needed and shake well before drinking.

Nutritional Information: Calories: 209, Total Fat: <1g, Saturated Fat: 0g, Protein: 1g, Carbohydrates: 56g, Fiber: 1g, Sodium: 25mg

Berry-Hibiscus Sports Drink

YIELD: Serves 1 **PREP TIME:** 5 to 10 minutes **COOK TIME:** 3 minutes

Hibiscus tea is floral in taste and can aid in digestion, fight inflammation, and stabilize blood sugar levels. This lightly sweetened sports drink is sure to hit the spot and provide a boost of antioxidants, glycogen, and electrolytes when you need them most.

12 ounces water

1 hibiscus tea bag, caffeine-free

2 tablespoons honey

⅛ teaspoon salt

4 strawberries, roughly chopped

1. In a microwave, in a microwave-safe mug or bowl, heat the water until boiling. Add the tea bag and let steep for 3 minutes or according to directions. Add in the honey and salt and stir until dissolved. Place the tea in a container and chill immediately.

2. Once the beverage is cool, add the strawberries and shake. Drink immediately or refrigerate for up to 6 hours.

Storage: Need your sports drink to last longer? Place in a freezer-friendly bottle or container and put directly in the freezer after mixing. Take out of the freezer at least 4 to 5 hours before needed and shake well before drinking.

Nutritional Information: Calories: 142, Total Fat: <1g, Saturated Fat: 0g, Protein: <1g, Carbohydrates: 38g, Fiber: 1g, Sodium: 180mg

Tart Cherry Sports Drink

YIELD: Serves 1 **PREP TIME:** 5 minutes **COOK TIME:** 1 minute

Tart cherry juice has been shown in some studies to reduce inflammation and muscle damage in athletes due to its antioxidants and high polyphenol count. If you're looking to delay fatigue and replenish glycogen, this sports drink recipe is for you.

12 ounces water, divided

¼ lime, juiced

⅛ teaspoon salt

8 ounces tart cherry juice, unsweetened

1. In a microwave, in a large microwave-safe cup or bowl, heat ½ cup of water and stir in the lime juice and salt. Stir until dissolved.

2. Add in the remaining 1 cup water and cherry juice. Serve immediately or chill in the fridge up to 1 day.

Storage: Need your sports drink to last longer? Place in a freezer-friendly bottle or container and put directly in the freezer after mixing. Take out of the freezer at least 4 hours before needed and shake well before drinking.

Nutritional Information: Calories: 143, Total Fat: 0g, Saturated Fat: 0g, Protein: 0g, Carbohydrates: 35g, Fiber: 0g, Sodium: 214mg

GLOSSARY

Aerobic: A term used to describe when oxygen is present.

Amenorrhea: The abnormal absence of a woman's menstrual cycle.

Anaerobic: A term used to describe when oxygen is not present.

Anorexia nervosa: A clinical diagnosis for an individual who has food avoidance and a skewed body image. Often manifests due to a fear of becoming overweight or obese.

Antioxidant: A compound that helps protect cells from free radical damage. Antioxidants can be found in a variety of fruits, vegetables, and whole grains.

Appetite: A desire for food, whether driven by emotion or physiological need.

Body Mass Index (BMI): A potential indicator of nutrition and health status calculated based on an individual's height and weight measurements. BMI does not take into account an individual's fat versus fat-free mass, and therefore is not an adequate determinant of health for athletes.

Bulimia nervosa: A clinical condition in which an individual experiences repeated bouts of binge-eating that are uncontrollable, and which leads to a large number of calories being eaten at a given time, followed by purging.

Complex carbohydrate: A carbohydrate composed of two or more simple sugar molecules.

Creatine monohydrate: A supplement that may be used to improve an athlete's strength and power when undergoing resistance exercise.

Dehydration: A condition that occurs when water loss exceeds water balance in an individual.

Dietary fiber: A form of carbohydrate obtained from plants that is indigestible by the body. Dietary fiber helps maintain proper digestion, and may improve cholesterol levels and regulate blood sugar.

Dietary supplement: A vitamin, mineral, herb, or other substance whose goal is not to serve as a main food source, but to supplement the diet in addition to one's food intake.

Digestion: A process in the body where food is broken down, and nutrients and energy are absorbed into the body.

Doping: The use of performance-enhancing substances, either artificially or through illegal measures.

Energy-yielding nutrients: Carbohydrates, proteins, and fats are nutrients that provide an energy source to the body. Also see macronutrients.

Fat-free mass: Primarily made up of skeletal muscle, protein, and organs. This is all the non-
fat-containing mass present in the body.

Fat mass: The amount of fat present in the body that makes up part of the overall body composition. This includes fat stored in cells as well as body fat.

Female Athlete Triad: Three health conditions that are diagnosed in female athletes, including disordered eating, menstrual irregularities or amenorrhea, and osteopenia or osteoporosis.

Fortified foods: Foods with added vitamins or minerals to their composition that were not
initially present.

Fructose: A simple sugar that is derived from fruits.

Glucose: The most common simple sugar present in carbohydrate-containing foods.

Glycogen: The storage form of glucose in the human body.

Macronutrients: Carbohydrates, protein, and fats. Also see energy-yielding nutrients.

Micronutrients: Nutrients needed by the body in trace amounts for health and functioning. Micronutrients include vitamins and minerals.

Phytochemicals: Plant-based chemicals present in fruits and vegetables, which have been shown to have health benefits for humans.

Prohormone: A substance that can be easily converted by the body into a biologically active hormone.

Registered dietitian: A nationally recognized nutrition expert. An individual who has passed the national registration examination for registered dietitians and is trained to provide nutrition education and counseling to the general public.

Satiety: A feeling of fullness that occurs after ingestion of food or beverages.

Starch: The storage form of carbohydrates present in plant-based foods. Starches consist of several chains of linked glucose molecules.

United States Anti-Doping Agency (USADA): An organization that serves as the U.S. branch of the World Anti-Doping Agency.

RESOURCES

EatRight Sports and Performance. The Academy of Nutrition and Diatetics: https://www.eatright.org/fitness#Sports-and-Performance

National Eating Disorders Association: https://www.nationaleatingdisorders.org/

NCAA 2019–2020 Banned Substances List: http://www.ncaa.org/sport-science-institute/topics/2019-20-ncaa-banned-substances

REFERENCES

Academy of Nutrition and Dietetics. Joint position statement. Nutrition and athletic performance. March 2016. Vol. 1 (16–93). 2016.

American Academy of Pediatrics. Promotion of healthy weight-control practices in youth athletes. *Pediatrics* 116(6): 1557–1564. 2005.

American College of Sports Medicine. Position stand paper: Exercise and fluid replacement. Medicine & Science in Sports Exercise. 377–389. 2007.

Aragon, A. A., and B. J. Schoenfeld. Nutrient timing revisited: Is there a post-exercise anabolic window? *Journal of the International Society of Sports Nutrition* 10(1): 5. 2013.

Baker, L. B., L. E. Heaton, R. P. Nuccio, et al. Dietitian-observed macronutrient intake of young skill and team-sport athletes: Adequacy of pre, during, and post exercise nutrition. *International Journal of Sport Nutrition and Exercise Metabolism* 24(2): 166–176. 2014.

Bar-Or, Oded. Nutritional considerations of the child athlete. *Canadian Journal of Applied Physiology* 26. 2001.

Bloodworth, A. J., et al. Doping and supplementation. The attitudes of talented young athletes. *Scandinavian Journal of Medicine and Science in Sports* 22(2): 293–301. 2012.

Boisseau, Natalie, Sonia Vera-Perez, and Jacques Poortmans. Food and fluid intake in adolescent female judo athletes before competition. *Pediatric Exercise Science* 17: 62–71. 2005.

Brown, G. A., et al. Testosterone prohormone supplements. *Medicine & Science in Sports & Exercise* 38(8): 1451–1461. 2006.

Burke, L. M., et al. Training and competition in nutrition. *Practical Sports Nutrition*. Human Kinetics. 2007.

Calfee, Ryan, and Paul Fadale. Popular ergogenic drugs and supplements in young athletes. *Pediatrics* 117: 577–588. 2006.

Casa, D., L. Armstrong, S. Maintain, B. Rich, et al. Physical activity levels to estimate the energy requirement of adolescent athletes. *Pediatric Exercise Science* 23: 261–269. 2011.

Connolly, D., et al. Efficacy of tart cherry juice blend in preventing the symptoms of muscle damage. *British Journal of Sports Medicine* 40(8): 679–683. 2006.

Council for Responsible Nutrition (CRN). The dietary supplement consumer. 2014. www.crnusa.org/CRN/consumer/survey.

Council for Responsible Nutrition. Guidelines for young athletes; Responsible use of sports nutrition supplements. 2002. www.crnusa.org.

Cribb P., A. Williams, and A. Hayes. A creatinine-protein-carbohydrate supplement enhances responses to resistance training. *Med Sci Sports Exercise* 39(11): 1960–1968. 2007.

Deminice, R., et al. Effects of creatine supplementation on oxidative stress and inflammation markers after repeated-sprint exercise in humans. *Nutrition* 29(9): 1127–1131. 2013.

Di Santolol, Manuela, Giuiana Stel, Giuseppe Banfi, et al. Anemia and iron status in young fertile non-professional female athletes. *European Journal of Applied Physiology* 102(6): 703–709. 2008.

Doherty, M., and P. Smith. Effects of caffeine ingestion on the rating of perceived exertion during and after exercise. A meta-analysis. *Scandinavian Journal of Medical Science and Sports*. 15(2): 69–78. 2005.

Etchison, W. C., E. A. Bloodgood, C. P. Minton, et al. Body mass index and percentage of body fat as indicators for obesity in an adolescent athletic population. *Sports Health* 3(3): 249–252. 2011.

Eudy, A. E. Efficacy and safety of ingredients found in pre-workout supplements. *American Journal of Health-System Pharmacy* 70(7): 577–588. 2013.

Fink, Heather Hendrick, Lisa A. Burgoon, and Alan E. Mikesky. *Practical Application in Sports Nutrition, 2nd Ed.* Jones and Bartlett. 155–188. 2008.

Fitzgerald, J. S., B. J. Peterson, J. M. Warpeha, et al. Association between vitamin D status and maximal-intensity exercise performance in junior and collegiate hockey players. *Journal of Strength and Conditioning Research* 29(9): 2513–2520. 2015.

Giesemer, B. A. Ergogenic risks elevate health risks in youth athletes. *Pediatric Annals* 32(11): 733–737. 2003.

Hoffman, Jay, et al. Nutritional supplementation and anabolic steroid use in adolescents. *Medicine & Science in Sports & Exercise* 40(1): 15–24. 2008.

Holway, F., and L. Spriet. Sport-specific nutrition: Practical strategies for team sports. *Journal of Sports Sciences* 29(1): 115–125. 2011.

Hoyte, C. O., et al. The use of energy drinks, dietary supplements, and prescription medications by United States college students to enhance athletic performance. *Journal of Community Health* 38(3): 575–580. 2013.

Jeukendrup, A. E. Carbohydrate and exercise performance. The role of multiple transportable carbohydrates. *Current Opinion in Clinical Nutrition and Metabolic Care* 13(4): 452–457. 2010.

Joy, Elizabeth, Mary Jane De Souza, Aurelia Nattiv, et al. Female athlete triad coalition consensus statement on treatment and return to play of the female athlete triad. *Current Sports Medicine Reports* 13(4): 219–232. 2014.

Lazar, Veronica, Lia-Mara Ditu, Gratiela Gradisteanu Pircalabioru, et al., "Aspects of Gut Microbiota and Immune System Interactions in Infection Diseases, Immunopathology, and Cancer." *Frontiers in Immunology* 9. 2018. https://doi.org/10.3389/fimmu.2018.01830.

Kong, P., and L. M. Harris. The sports body: Body image and eating disorder symptoms among female athletes from leanness focused and nonleanness focused sports. *Journal of Psychology* 149(1): 141–160. 2015.

Mamerow, M., J. Mettler, K. English, et al. Dietary protein distribution positively influences 24-h muscle protein synthesis in healthy adults. *Journal of Nutrition* 144(6): 876–880. 2014.

Matzkin, E., E. J. Curry, and K. Whitlock. Female athlete triad: Past, present and future. *Journal of the American Academy of Orthopedic Surgeons* 23(7): 424–432. 2015.

Mettler, S., N. Mitchell, and K. Tipton. Increased protein intake reduces lean body mass loss during weight loss in athletes. *Medicine & Science in Sports & Exercise* 42(2): 326–337. 2010.

Milewski, M. D., D. L. Skaggs, G. A. Bishop, et al. Chronic lack of sleep is associated with increased sports injuries in adolescent athletes. *Journal of Pediatric Orthopedics* 34(2): 129–133. 2014.

National Institutes of Health. National Institutes of Health state-of-the-science conference statement: Multi-vitamins and mineral supplements and chronic disease prevention. *American Journal of Clinical Nutrition* 85(1): 257–264. 2007.

Pasiakos, S. M., J. J. Cao, L. M. Margolis, et al. Effects of high-protein diets on fat free mass and muscle protein synthesis following weight loss: A randomized controlled trial. *FASEB Journal* 27(9): 3837–3847. 2013.

Philips, S., and L. Van Loon. Dietary protein for athletes: From requirements to optimum adaptation. *Journal of Sports Science* 29(1): 29–38. 2011.

Reed, S. C., F. Levin, and S. Evans. Changes in mood, cognitive performance and appetite in the late luteal and follicular phases of the menstrual cycle in women with and without PMDD. *Hormonal Behavior* 54(1): 185–193. 2008.

Rosenbloom, Christine, et al. *Sports Nutrition: A Practical Manual for Professionals, 5th ed.* Academy of Nutrition and Dietetics. 2012.

Spaccarotella, K. J., and W. D. Andzel. The effects of low-fat chocolate milk on postexercise recovery in collegiate athletes. *Journal of Strength and Conditioning Research* 25(12): 3456–3460. 2011.

Stellingwerff, T., R. Maughan, and L. Burke. Nutrition for power sports: Middle-distance running, track, cycling, rowing, canoeing, kayaking, and swimming. *Journal of Sports Sciences* 29(1): 79–89. 2011.

Tokmakidis, S. P., and I. A. Karamanolis. Effects of carbohydrate ingestion 15 minutes before exercise on endurance running capacity. *Applied Physiology, Nutrition and Metabolism* 33(3): 441–448. 2008.

Torun, Benjamin. Energy requirements of children and adolescents. *Public Health Nutrition* 8(7A), 968–993. 2005.

U.S. Department of Health and Human Services. 2015–2020 Dietary Guidelines for Americans, 8th ed. 2015. http://health.gov/dietaryguidelines/2015/guidelines.

Weiss, Alison, Fang Xu, Amy Starfer-Isser, et al. The association of sleep duration with adolescents' fat and carbohydrate consumption. *Sleep* 33(9): 1201–1209. 2010.

INDEX

ACKNOWLEDGMENTS

Thank you to my friends and family, who not only challenged me to pursue this project but cheered me on every step of the way. This project would not have been as much fun without you. A special thank you to Gabriel, who was there every day for me during this process. Thank you for listening, encouraging me, and dealing with my extremely erratic schedule without a single complaint. I love and appreciate you more than you'll ever know.

ABOUT THE AUTHOR

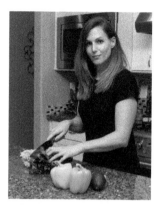

Jackie Slomin, MS, RDN, is an internationally recognized sports nutritionist, registered dietitian, and author with a master's degree in sports nutrition and exercise science. Jackie has worked with hundreds of athletes to show them how to increase strength, gain a competitive edge, and reach body composition and weight goals. She works with athletes of all shapes and sizes but specializes in helping high school– and college-aged wrestlers make weight and break performance barriers on and off the mat without aggressive weight-cutting techniques. There are a number of free resources available on www.jackieslomin.com and www.nutritiononthemat.com that athletes can use for further help achieving peak performance through sports nutrition.

9 781646 117093